Nursing and Health Care
Research

PRENTICE HALL NURSING SERIES

A series of comprehensive textbooks and reference manuals for nurses and other health care professionals.

Other titles in the series include:

Teaching and Assessing in Clinical Nursing Practice
edited by Peter L. Bradshaw

Clinical Nursing Manual
edited by Jennifer E. Clark

Legal Aspects of Nursing, second edition
Bridgit Dimond

Nursing Care of Women
Dinah Gould

Drugs and Nursing Implications
Laura E. Govoni and Janice E. Hayes (adapted by Jill A. David)

Research and Statistics: A Practical Introduction for Nurses
Carolyn M. Hicks

Becoming a Staff Nurse: A Guide to the Role of the Newly Registered Nurse
edited by Judith Lathlean and Jessica Corner

Nursing Concepts for Health Promotion
Ruth Beckman Murray and Judith Proctor Zentner (adapted by Cindy Howells)

Body Image: Nursing Concepts and Care
Bob Price

Clinical Nursing Practice: The Promotion and Management of Continence
Brenda Roe

The Art and Science of Midwifery
Louise Silverton

Nursing the Patient with Cancer, second edition
edited by Verena Tschudin

Nursing and Health Care Research

A Skills-based Introduction

Second edition

Collette Clifford

PRENTICE HALL
LONDON   NEW YORK   TORONTO   SYDNEY   TOKYO
SINGAPORE   MADRID   MEXICO CITY   MUNICH   PARIS

First published in 1990 by
Prentice Hall International (UK) Ltd
as *Nursing Research: a skills-based introduction*
edited by Collette Clifford and Stephen Gough
This edition published 1997 by
Prentice Hall Europe
Campus 400, Maylands Avenue
Hemel Hempstead
Hertfordshire, HP2 7EZ
A division of
Simon & Schuster International Group

© Prentice Hall International (UK) Ltd, 1990; Prentice Hall Europe, 1997

Typeset in 10/12 Times
by PPS, London Road, Amesbury, Wiltshire

Printed and bound in Great Britain by
Redwood Books, Trowbridge, Wiltshire

Library of Congress Cataloging-in-Publication Data

Clifford, Collette
    Nursing and health care research : a skills-based introduction /
Collette Clifford. – 2nd ed.
        p.   cm. – (Prentice Hall nursing series)
    Includes bibliographical references and index.
    ISBN 0–13–229741–8
    1. Nursing–Research.   2. Medical care–Research.   I. Title.
II. Series.
    [DNLM: 1. Nursing Research–methods.   2. Health Services Research-
–methods.   WY 20.5 C637n 1997]
    RT81.5.C53   1997
    610.73'072–dc21
    DNLM/DLC
    for Library of Congress   96-37311
                                                                          CIP

British Library Cataloguing in Publication Data

A catalogue record for this book is available from
the British Library

ISBN: 0–13–229741–8

---

1 2 3 4 5   01 00 99 98 97

Contents

Introduction to the second edition

When the first edition of this book was developed, the perceived need was to approach research from the perspective of the newcomer to research. The aim of the text was to 'keep it simple' and avoid tangling the issues in jargon that might cause confusion. This aim remains the same in this second edition, which has been expanded to explore the research process in greater depth whilst, at the same time, retaining a text that is readily accessible to nursing and health care practitioners who, for whatever reason, want to know more about research. This includes those who may be involved in developing small-scale clinically based projects at diploma to degree level and those more experienced researchers who want a resource for some aspects of the research process.

The development of a number of sections in the second edition of this book serves perhaps as an indication of the changes that have occurred in health care education and research over recent years. Whilst the first edition met the needs of newcomers to research at that time it is no longer sufficient to meet the needs of the nurse and health care professionals as we move towards the year 2000. Research studies are now an integral part of the curriculum in educational programmes and health care practitioners are expected to be more actively involved in the research process from the point of developing ideas, initiating enquiry to disseminating and implementing research to ensure the optimal outcome of care. The emphasis of this text, as in the first edition, is to trace the research process from the initial idea through to dissemination and implementation of findings as appropriate. In so doing, a number of sections have been enlarged and updated. This includes a greater emphasis on some of the 'planning' issues in research seen as particularly important given the increased opportunity available for practitioners to take part in funded research projects. From this perspective increased emphasis has been given to acquiring funding for research and working with established systems of ethical approval.

The increasing interest in qualitative approaches to research in health care is reflected in an exploration of knowledge development in health care and the use of qualitative approaches in data collection and analysis. The sections exploring quantitative methods have been expanded to meet the needs of health care practitioners who might be involved in undertaking small-scale projects in clinical practice.

The last chapters focus on dissemination and implementation of research. The chapter on writing for research has been expanded to meet the needs of practitioners at different stages of the research process, again starting 'at the beginning' with basic writing skills and working through a range of skills related to writing for research up to the point of publication of research. The last chapter briefly outlines some of the strategic issues that are influencing the development of health care research today and focuses on a few key issues of relevance to the utilisation research in practice.

Overall, in increasing the range of skills explored in this text, it is hoped that this text will be a useful guide to the research process and a resource text for those who wish to use the text more selectively, perhaps to help the practitioner who is developing the skills required to read published research reports critically.

Whilst recognising the risks involved in writing for an audience beyond one's own professional group, an attempt has been made to make the text accessible to a wider audience of health care practitioners. Although I must take the ultimate responsibility for any apparent inconsistencies that are evident in the examples which seek to give a range of perspectives, I am very grateful for the help and advice given by a small group of professional colleagues who have reviewed the text and made helpful suggestions. Ros Carnwell, Sarah Murray and Ros Grant examined the draft version of the text from the differing perspectives of community health, acute nursing and physiotherapy. They undertook this task with great willingness and offered no word of complaint about the effort involved in undertaking this review. However, I was very much aware of the time and personal effort involved in this and wish to express my gratitude to them all.

Collette Clifford 1996

Introduction to the first edition

The overall content of this book is based on several years of experience of introducing nursing staff and student nurses to research. The framework is one that has been used with some success in motivating interest in research at an introductory level. The emphasis given to each issue identified in the book reflects areas of uncertainty that have caused particular difficulties for nurses approaching research studies for the first time.

The first chapter gives a general introduction to the topic. In focusing on the 'what, why and who' in nursing research it is hoped that newcomers to the subject may gain insight into the wider issues involved in developing research skills in nursing. The second chapter focuses on research awareness. This is seen to be an important inclusion in an introductory text for study of nursing research that does not necessarily mean undertaking a research project. The aim of a course of study in research may be to enhance awareness of research in general.

The next three chapters focus on the research process. Chapter 3 concentrates on generating research ideas. Nurses approaching research studies for the first time often have more difficulty with this than with any other aspect of the research process. This is followed by a chapter on some of the general practical issues involved in planning research.

Chapter 5 outlines the research process and offers a source of reference for the process as a whole. The outline in this chapter could also be useful for nurses who are learning to read research literature critically, for it offers a framework by which research reports can be analysed.

The chapter on literature searching is the only chapter not written exclusively for newcomers. The comprehensive explanation of how to search literature and the resources available to help nurses in this provides a useful source of reference for anyone involved in research studies.

In examining approaches to research and the methods and techniques deployed in data collection Chapter 7 gives quite a wide range of information. Each of the areas discussed in this chapter could, and do, provide enough material for books in their own right and so the limitations of this chapter are recognised. However, the content reflects the issues that cause concern to nurses approaching research studies at an elementary level and it is not intended for it be a definitive guide on data collection. A short chapter on analysing research data has been included to help nurses understand some of the techniques used by researchers to analyse and present data. This is felt to be important as familiarity with some of the issues identified in Chapter 8 will do much to enhance understanding of research reports using statistical techniques to present data.

Sharing knowledge is a crucial part of research studies. It has been common practice in our school, in common with many others, to place much emphasis on this component as part of research studies. However, it has been our experience that preparation of written material related to research has caused considerable anxiety to those nurses expected to write essays on research, research proposals or research reports. In addition, the presentation of information gained through research studies can, and does, cause extreme anxiety to newcomers to nursing research. Consequently, although a chapter on presentation skills is not common in texts on research we see this as an important inclusion in this book. Both aspects have formed part of programmes of research studies, for the sharing of research knowledge is crucial if we are to enhance the professional knowledge base.

As knowledge of research increases so the need to change practices may be identified. Consequently, in the final chapter, the use of change theory has been included to help those nurses who wish to introduce research-based practices into their own area of work.

Because of the variety of material explored in this book each chapter stands alone as a source of reference. There are areas of overlap as some issues identified in earlier chapters are examined in more depth in later sections. Where this occurs the reader is referred to other relevant sections of the book.

In any introductory text the range and depth of material examined is, of necessity, limited. A list of further reading is given at the end of each chapter as a means of overcoming this problem.

It can be seen that in taking a skills-based approach to an introduction to nursing research the emphasis in this book extends beyond the skills required to undertake research in nursing. Other issues seen as important to nurses in the developing and sharing knowledge of research have been explored. The content of the book reflects specific areas identified as causing anxiety by nurses who are beginning studies of research and consequently it is anticipated that it will be a useful reference text for those in this position.

Within this text, in the interest of uniformity of approach, the female pronoun 'she' is used throughout to refer to the nurse.

1   Research for health care

The interest in research in health care has grown rapidly in recent years to the extent that all health care professionals are now encouraged to ensure that their practices reflect knowledge based on research rather than practices determined by tradition.

In this chapter three aspects of research are explored:

1. Research for health care practitioners.
2. Why research is required in health care.
3. Who can be involved in research in health care.

What is research in health care?

As the interest in research in health care has grown, the number of definitions and explorations of the topic has increased. Most definitions of research follow a similar theme with the search for knowledge being emphasised as a fundamental reason for undertaking research studies. There is a general consensus that this search must follow a *'logical planned format'* for it to be classed as a research study. This logical planned process distinguishes research from other types of project that may be undertaken for the purpose of enquiry.

This is important in health care for there are many different formats that may be used when undertaking enquiries. For example a new health care student may undertake a project to determine the health education facilities available in his or her district. At the early stage of a course it would not be normally expected for this student to have an extensive knowledge of the research process or techniques of data collection. Consequently the means by which the student collects information will be left very much to his or her own initiative and so the teacher may expect a variety of approaches to be used by students.

Further analysis of a number of definitions of research show similar themes emerging through all of them. The emphasis in each varies but, in general terms, there is some note made of research reflecting a *scientific* process. The word 'scientific' perhaps serves to make research appear to be somewhat distant from some aspects of health care practice. The associations with science may be seen as something more common to those used to working in laboratories rather than to people working with others in a health care setting.

The scientific approach to research indicates a situation in which there is 'control' over the factors that are being studied. By exerting this control, the researcher is attempting to predict what will happen following a planned sequence of activities. In using such an approach the researcher is in fact using the principle of an experimental research design, which we will return to later in this text.

Although the notion of doing an experiment is familiar to many of us, it does represent quite a complex approach to research. This can easily be illustrated in relation to our own experiences. In a laboratory setting in our school days we may have done experiments by mixing a little of substance 'A' with a little of substance 'B' and produced substance 'C'. If this was done on ten occasions, and if each occasion produced the same result, then we would feel fairly confident that on the eleventh occasion the same result would occur. In other words we would be predicting the outcome based on the findings of our experiment.

If using an experimental approach to health care research the researcher will approach the study in a similar controlled way. The goal of the research would be to predict the outcome of a given situation based on the findings of the experimental study. All factors should be monitored closely and the pattern of events analysed to determine the outcome on each occasion.

There are very practical uses for this type of research in health care but, when studying people, it is not so easy to have control over all of the variables involved in the experiment in the same way as it is in the laboratory when working with chemical substances.

For example, the nurse searching for the perfect technique to enhance healing of the infected wound may choose to carry out an experimental study to determine which is the most effective wound dressing to use in this situation. She would need to consider a large number of variables including factors such as age, wound site, causative organisms, other underlying diseases and so on. The benefits of such research are that a nurse might then be able to predict with some confidence that a particular dressing was the one most likely to promote a quick recovery in her patients with wound infection.

In experimental studies such as this there are specific requirements in terms of being able to 'manipulate' the substance being studied (in this case the wound dressing) and therefore to control the situation being studied. Because of the complexity of this there is not a long tradition of experimental research in some branches of health care including nursing and other health care workers such as physiotherapists, midwives, occupational therapists and so on. This contrasts with medical research which relies heavily on the experimental approach to determine the effectiveness of new treatment particularly, for example, for new drug therapies. Consequently alternative approaches to research, which do not seek to predict outcomes, have been more commonly utilised by a wide range of health workers. Rather than attempting to exert control in an experimental situation, for example, the researcher may analyse the relationship between observed events in an approach to research known as *correlational research design*, may compare two sets of results – *comparative research design* – or may simply observe and describe what is happening – *descriptive research*. We will look at these different designs in more detail later in the text.

Whichever approach is taken to research, the common themes to emerge in any definitions of research is that *'research is a planned, logical process. Research may be undertaken for the purpose of analysing relationships between events, or for predicting outcomes.'*

Research may be seen as a problem-solving process undertaken in the pursuit of knowledge. The 'problem' is the area that is the subject of the study whether that be the value of particular wound dressing in an experimental study or, in a correlational study or an account of what is observed in a descriptive study, the pattern of events in a food poisoning outbreak. In determining the problem area, the researcher would be very specific in stating the area of enquiry when planning a study.

Some types of research may not have a clearly defined 'problem' area at the outset. In the pursuit of knowledge the researcher may look for understanding, or meaning, in a given situation; for example, what it means to be a health care student. This approach does not identify a 'problem' for research, but rather seeks to add to the body of knowledge by taking an in-depth look at one particular situation, by trying to understand the meaning. We will discuss this later when we examine qualitative approaches to research.

In summary, research can be seen as a search for knowledge in which the format of the enquiry is logical and clearly defined. A variety of approaches to research can be identified, and each should be utilised appropriately in relation to the subject of enquiry.

Why research in health care?

An increasing number of health care professionals are resolving their own uncertainties about research by undertaking research appreciation courses in which their insight and knowledge of the subject can be increased. However, there are still many practitioners who see research as something new and consequently tend to view it with suspicion. It is recognised that this suspicion may come from uncertainty about what research means, and what the implications of using research are to health care practitioners. Although there is increasing knowledge about the subject among practitioners there remains an element of mystique associated with the research process and it is this that I hope to dispel in this book.

The reason for uncertainty about research lies in the history of the health care professions. From a nursing perspective it is interesting to note that Florence Nightingale is frequently given credit in many research texts for being the first nurse researcher. The statistical work she produced to support her arguments for the developing nursing workforce in the early days of organised nursing should be reviewed by any potential recruits to research. It was perhaps unfortunate that in her time Miss Nightingale did not identify the value of encouraging others to take such an analytic approach to their work, concentrating instead upon the practicalities of doing nursing. As the origins of the therapy professions can be traced back to the origins of nursing, many of the issues that influenced the evolution of these professions can be allied to nursing. Even those professions that have older roots than nursing, such as midwifery, were influenced by developments in nursing as they were allied to nursing for the purpose of regulation and control of professional development in the twentieth century.

A key factor to consider was the location of professional training in schools located in the UK National Health Service (NHS), unlike medical education which was developing in the university sector, the location of research activity. Professional education located in the NHS emphasised doing 'the tasks', whilst education in the university sector focused on the thought processes behind the 'task' and encouraged people to ask the question '*why*?'. As you will see later the word 'why' underpins research activity.

Over the years changes to the educational programmes for all health care professionals have resulted in the development of academic departments of health and nursing in the university sector in the United Kingdom. This means that all health care professional groups are now located in the university sector and are in a strong position to develop their educational base and thus research. These educational changes have been accompanied by many other changes at individual professional level. For example changes in the demographic distribution of members of health care groups have resulted in an increase in women entering the profession of medicine and men choosing nursing and other allied professions as their career. This will impact on research as some will suggest that the gender of researchers can influence the way in which research is developed. This may be reviewed further from the literature on *feminist research.*

The other major change that has, and will continue to have, a major influence on health care research is the major reorganisation of health care provision in the United Kingdom and the pressure from government to ensure that practices in health care are based on a sound knowledge base rather than ritualistic or traditional practices. In the United Kingdom in the 1990s the Department of Health (DoH) has established a major initiative to ensure that research for practice is well co-ordinated and developed to meet the needs of health care. The research and development (R&D) strategy for the NHS was established in 1991 and is now an integral part of health care management. The impact of this strategy can now be seen from the DoH level down to practice where the key question in health care is 'what is the outcome of this treatment; is it effective?'. The responses generated by such questions have served to challenge health care practices developed over many years and to identify wide variation in approaches across the United Kingdom and wider. In the face of this challenge health care practitioners can no longer ignore the centrality of research in practice.

Who is involved in research in health care?

There are an increasing number of jobs in health care in which research is picked out as a key area of responsibility. Increasingly, however, a research component is being included in many job descriptions for professionals involved in health care.

In the light of the NHS R&D strategy the answer to the question of who can do research is any practitioner, at any level of practice. However, as you will see later in the book it may not be appropriate to talk of who can do research; rather we should be considering who might use research. Indeed a major thrust of the NHS R&D strategy is that of developing a system of review and dissemination to support practitioners who do not have the time or scope to do research.

Throughout this text applied examples will be related to many areas of practice to illustrate the points made. No single group of practitioners is confined to an area of interest, and research in health care practice includes not only clinical practice, but also management and education for practice. Increasingly the emphasis in health care research is on multi-disciplinary, collaborative projects in which care is examined from a variety of perspectives.

At a practice level, the practitioner is well placed to carry out clinical care research projects, whilst at management level the manager may choose to vary the emphasis in any research into care and consider the effects of any research-based changes in managing the unit. Finally lecturers in health care may be interested to examine the impact of teaching on the quality of care produced by students. These examples indicate very briefly the range of subject areas that could be incorporated under the title of health care research. Add to this the study of 'care' itself, which has provided a focus not only for health care practitioners but also for many other disciplines such as sociologists and psychologists, and the area of research in health care becomes even wider.

Before moving from this section it is worth emphasising one point that has relevance for all readers – whilst all health care practitioners can do research, it would not be appropriate for all to do so. In contrast all health care workers should be able to use research. To do so, however, requires understanding about what is involved in research – research awareness, which we will review in the next chapter.

ACTIVITY _____

Consider your own professional background and the point at which you were first introduced to research:

- Was this introduced positively?
- Were you clear about the purpose of research for your own discipline?
- Did you understand the process involved?
- Try to define research in the context of your own discipline.

Summary

This chapter has briefly explored definitions of research and considered why we need research in health care. The issue of who can do research has been briefly addressed and the use of research-based practices in the context of clinical practice, management or education outlined.

Further reading

Abbott, P. and Sapsford, R. (1992) *Research Methods for Nurses and the Caring Professions*, Open University Press, Buckingham.

Altshull, A. (1991) 'The development of research in nursing', in Cormack, D. F. S., *The Research Process in Nursing*, 2nd edn, Blackwell Scientific Publications, Oxford, Ch. 2.

Chapman, J. (1991) 'Research – What it is and what it is not', in Perry, A. and Jolley, M., *Nursing – A Knowledge Base for Practice*, Edward Arnold, London, Ch. 2.

Clark, E. (1991) *Research Awareness Module 3 What is Research?* Distance Learning Centre, South Bank Polytechnic (South Bank University), London.

Clifford, C., Carnwell, R. and Harkin, L. (1996) *Research Methodology in Nursing and Health Care*, Open Learning Foundation/Churchill Livingstone, Edinburgh.

Hockey, L. (1985) *Nursing Research – Mistakes and Misconceptions*, Churchill Livingstone, Edinburgh.

Jolley, M. (1993) 'Out of the past', in Jolley, M. and Brykczñska, G., *Nursing, its Hidden Agendas*, Edward Arnold, London, Ch. 1.

Reed, J. and Proctor, S. (Eds) (1995) *Practitioner Research in Health Care: The Inside Story*, Chapman & Hall, London.

Webb, C. (1993) 'Feminist research: definitions, methodology, methods and evaluation', *Journal of Advanced Nursing*, Vol. 18, no. 30, pp. 416–423.

2   Research awareness

The purpose of this chapter is to explore some of the general issues that have an impact on the ability of health care practitioners to use research in their practice. In the previous chapter it was suggested that not all practitioners will be or should be active researchers. By this it was meant that not all would go out and collect data using the systematic process of research outlined earlier. Indeed if all practitioners were to do this it would create major problems in health care as such a scenario would mean that perhaps all patients or clients requiring care would be expected to participate in research, which is not an ideal situation. However, as indicated earlier, all health care practitioners should incorporate research-based knowledge into their practice. To do this they need to be research aware, to know how to access and use research in practice. From this perspective we will begin to consider specific skills required in research in this chapter and focus on the skills related to research awareness. This includes a review of the following:

1. Factors affecting research awareness.
2. Research and knowledge of research.
3. Utilising research awareness in practice.

In placing the emphasis on research awareness at this early stage in the book it is hoped that readers will realise that research-based practice is not just about doing research, it is also about being aware of the availability of research and utilising research-based knowledge in practice at every opportunity. This leads to using research and finally to considering ways in which health care practitioners can share research experiences with each other through systems of dissemination of research in health care.

Research awareness

The term 'research awareness' is frequently used to denote what some may see as a special kind of skill. In fact it is a useful term to cover all levels of interest in research. Although not all nurses and other health care practitioners will be researchers, all should be aware of research and have sufficient knowledge of this to utilise research in their practice.

To be aware of research implies that the practitioner has an understanding of the principles of research and has sufficient knowledge to read and analyse research reports critically. Research awareness means being prepared to ask questions and to look for answers. To be aware of research means that the practitioner knows about the research that has been carried out in his or her own area of professional practice and utilises that knowledge in planning care or managing practice.

In summary, research awareness means that nurses or other health care professionals have an insight into the research process, are questioning in their approach to care, are familiar with research relevant to their practice and use that knowledge in their work.

Factors affecting research awareness

There are several reasons why research may be seen to be something separate from, rather than an integral part of, everyday clinical practice. The first reason for limited awareness of research amongst a range of health care professionals is historical. One area that may be seen to have a direct bearing on the development of research awareness in nursing and other health care professionals is linked to the models of education. For example, medical staff were educated in universities and so 'did research' whilst other health care professionals were educated in the NHS and so were trained to do the practical work necessary for care. New drugs and new surgical techniques were tried and tested before any doctor would say with confidence that the prescription for care would work. In contrast nurses and others were developing skill in 'caring' which is not so easy to assess in terms of impact. Whilst the impact of new surgical techniques, say for example key hole surgery, can be seen immediately in physiological terms, it is less easy to observe the result of care given by other members of the health care team.

The end result of this is that, whereas the medical profession can trace the origins of their research back several hundred years, the evolution of research for other health care workers in the United Kingdom has a much more recent history dating back to the 1950s and early 1960s. Nurses and other paramedical disciplines were not unused to research prior to that time, but rather they were accustomed to their medical colleagues undertaking research and so saw this as something separate from their practice. Nurses, for example, did, and still do, participate in medical research but the capacity in which this is done is more often that of a research assistant than as the initiator of research ideas. For example nurses may distribute drugs prescribed for a medically led drug trial (sometimes referred to as *clinical trials*), collect specimens for analysis following this or work as research assistants to medical research projects.

It is important, however, that the liaison with medical practice is not seen as the sole reason for the failure of nurses and others to develop research awareness at an earlier stage in the evolution of the profession. Other factors outlined below have had an impact and will be explored in relation to this.

Ritual, intuition or knowledge-based practice?

When we refer to 'knowledge-based practice' we mean that practitioners are using the most recent knowledge available to them to help direct and guide their practice. As research is about generating knowledge we could also refer to this as 'research-based' practice. When considering the topic of research awareness and the issue of research in practice we need to make a distinction between what we 'know' through research and what we 'know' through other forms of knowledge generation (Robinson and Vaughan 1992). Into such debates come issues related to patterns of behaviour that have become rituals as a result of years of routine practice. Another influencing factor, intuition, has also been criticised.

One of the criticisms commonly directed at health care practitioners is that the care given is adopted simply on the basis of preference of the practitioners rather than any sound knowledge base. The influence of those responsible for developing practical skills in the next generation of practitioners is such that it is not uncommon for a junior health care worker to adopt practices accepted as the preference of their seniors as being the 'right' way that things should be done. Such developments are commonly described as 'ritualistic' or 'traditional' practices; they are done simply because they have always been done that way. Now, whilst this is associated with long-standing patterns of practice, it should be noted that it does not take long for one approach to care to become 'ritualistic'.

You may be able to identify a number of areas depending on your professional background. For example, trainee midwives may have noted the long-standing habits of treating the umbilical cord in a variety of ways depending on the preference of the midwife; physiotherapists may have noted a shift away from intensive respiratory therapy for chronic respiratory problems; nurses may have noted how different ward sisters or charge nurses had different preferences for treating wounds; medical students may have noted that different surgeons have different preferences for the post-operative care despite the fact that both have performed the same surgical procedure. Most of these practices may have evolved on the basis of the preference of one person and so become a ritualistic way of practice rather than a knowledge-based practice. The lack of research in some aspects of care may have contributed to this but, as you will see in Chapter 5 this is not the only reason.

Another aspect that has often been criticised is 'intuition', which cannot claim practice is based on evident 'factual knowledge' but may be described as a 'gut feeling' that, in a given situation, something is not quite right. Many practitioners will relate to this: for example, many experienced nurses will tell of how they went back to check a patient because they simply 'felt' there was something wrong, to find that the patient needed urgent care. When asked to give reasons for going back to the patient the nurse might find it hard to explain, yet recognise that a 'gut feeling' was an inadequate explanation. Consequently, over the years the aspect of intuitive practice in nursing has provided a challenge for researchers who are now trying to unravel exactly what does happen when the nurse gets an intuition that all is not as it should be (see, for example, Benner 1987).

Research does not deny the individual instincts that practitioners have developed in the course of their careers, but rather it seeks to identify the foundation of that intuition so that the knowledge base for practice can be clarified. It must be acknowledged that just because something has always worked in one way before it does not mean that it will always work in that way on every occasion. For example, a car driver will have had the experience of assuming that when the key is turned in the ignition the engine will start. This may be the case on most occasions but one day the expected response may not occur: the key is turned and nothing happens. If the driver has some knowledge of mechanics he or she may be able to work out systematically what is wrong with the car and perhaps be able to fix the fault. If he or she is not able to do this, specialist help must be called in.

To use this as an analogy it may be suggested that the practitioner finds that on most occasions a given form of care, based on ritualistic or intuitive practices, works. However, on the occasions that the expected response does not occur, a practitioner with a sound knowledge base may review the alternatives, look for a solution to this particular problem and aim to solve it. If he or she does not have the appropriate knowledge then the subsequent result may be an incorrect solution, which may mean that the patient/client does not receive the appropriate care for their problem. Unfortunately the practitioner may not be in a position to call in the 'rescue services' as any one of us would be if our car broke down. There may be experts at hand in the form of specialists who have developed a research-based approach to their work. However, the practitioner steeped in ritualistic approaches may treat with mistrust those who have a role that is not conducive to traditional practice. Consequently he or she may not be prepared to call for further advice at a time of need.

One way in which it is possible for practitioners to explore the level of ritual or intuition in their own practice is to stop and ask themselves *why* they are carrying out care in a particular fashion. This is certainly a better way of approaching care than waiting for something to go wrong before seeking help. Also, as noted above, questioning practice serves to enhance research awareness and may facilitate the practitioner in identifying a clearly defined knowledge base to his or her work. .

Common sense

Common sense is a term that is frequently used to try to explain why we do something or, perhaps more frequently, to question why someone else did not do something! There is an assumption that, in many instances, the way things are done reflects a common bonding of ideas and approaches to a problem and that the subsequent method used to solve the problem will be common to all. We all think we know what 'common sense' means but unfortunately, as with many other aspects of life, what we think it means and what others think it means are not always the same. In other words common sense is not so common! Consequently, assumptions that care should be based on common sense are questionable for they can put the patient or client at risk.

It is appropriate to consider how practitioners gain knowledge of research as a subject for, although there is a growing awareness of research generally there are still many aspects that cause concern to nurses and other health care professionals interested in the utilisation of research findings.

Research and knowledge of research

As noted above, the history of research for health care workers is relatively recent, covering a span of approximately thirty years in the United Kingdom. This has had an impact on the development of knowledge of research in clinical practice.

Traditional patterns of education for nurses and other health care workers did not prepare them to be questioning and critical in their approach. In leading a more questioning approach to practice, the efforts of the early nurse researchers, for example, were important in that these practitioners began to scrutinise what was happening in their profession. This in turn eventually contributed towards a redirection in education programmes, although it was to take some years before research studies were an integral part of the curriculum. Consequently research into health care remained distant from the everyday practice of the majority of practitioners, tending to be located in institutes of higher education. The time taken for this research knowledge to cascade from higher education to the NHS education sector serves to explain why so many qualified practitioners remain uncertain about utilising research in their work. They simply did not have opportunity to study the topic of research when preparing for their initial qualification. This has changed now of course, but it is only since the mid to late 1980s that research has been an integral component of professional education and so, it must be stressed, this is only a recent innovation. The introduction of a research-orientated approach into education for health care professionals has been a slow process. The result of this is a deficit in all health care professions of people with an appropriate knowledge base to support research development in practice.

It should be noted that the key people involved in teaching research are of course the teachers or lecturers in various health care disciplines. There are many teachers of nursing who themselves had to learn about research before they could confidently teach the subject to students. Many of these teachers were themselves educated in the traditional mode in which research as a subject was not part of the syllabus.

Two further issues can be seen as directly linked with education for research. These are the ability of nurses and other health workers to understand the research information presented to them and the wider issue of the availability of research.

Understanding research

The ability of nurses and other health care workers to understand research links directly with education for if this was not adequate they will continue to have difficulty in understanding the purpose and value of research. It must be acknowledged that, although there are increasing numbers of health care students studying research, either through formal courses or self-directed study, there is still a need to consider ways in which individual understanding of research can be enhanced.

One area that is frequently cited as causing a difficulty to those wishing to understand more about research is the style of presentation of research reports. Frequently the presentation of information does not meet the needs of those people for whom it is intended – that is the rank and file of practitioners. There are several reasons seen as contributing to this. The use of 'jargon' is commonly noted as a factor that makes it difficult to understand research reports. This is not an intentional ploy on the part of the researchers, rather it indicates that very often published research has been undertaken as part of an academic study. The language used commonly reflects the 'academic' requirement but, while easily understood by those initiated into the rigours of academic life, it is not so comprehensible to those who have not had that experience.

Researchers themselves are well aware of this problem and some attempt to overcome it by writing their reports in two formats, the first for academic presentation and the second, a summarised version, for a more general readership. In the past there was a tendency for some people to disagree with researchers taking a dual approach when presenting their research findings and to argue that if the standard of research is to be maintained, then so the type of presentation should be consistent. However, a direct result of the recent drive to increase research utilisation within the NHS has been a clear effort to make sure that research reports presented are readily accessible to the market that will be using the results.

Since the early 1990s it has become much more common practice for researchers to produce a synopsis of their research findings in a short, easy-to-read fashion. A good example of this can be found in the series of publications produced by the English National Board for Nursing, Midwifery and Health Visiting, in which the full report is available for all, whilst an easy-to-read synopsis identifying the key finding of the research is available in the 'Research Highlights' series available from the Board. Not only is this an example of good practice but it is also an example of an organisational response to research which identified the problems encountered by practitioners who wish to access research findings without struggling through complex reports.

Another aspect that frequently acts as a deterrent to practitioners reading research reports is the use of statistical tables. As will be seen in Chapter 8, the use of statistical data in research reports is used to support and explain the information given by the researcher in the text. If practitioners have only an elementary knowledge of statistics they will find the inclusion of this data beneficial when reading research reports. Very often data that can be confusing on first review are not so complex once the reader has a basic understanding of research.

Library resources

Access to a good library is crucial if research awareness is to be developed. This factor has been recognised and many centres are now developing excellent library resources for health studies students. Issues that librarians have had to consider include not only the library resources available but also how to offer a flexible service to meet the needs of their area. This is important for nurses and health care professionals, as a group, are disparate in both their knowledge bases and their abilities to match their working hours to the opening hours of the library. There are many initiatives taking place at a local level in an attempt to meet these needs. Flexible opening hours is one example that can be used to illustrate this point.

All newcomers to research would be well advised to familiarise themselves with their local library and to use the skills offered by the librarian when developing their knowledge base of research. This is important for the rapid growth of computer technology has in the past few years revolutionised the way in which we can search for information for use in research.

Availability of research

The discussion above does appear to presume the availability of research. It is quite feasible that a practitioner may seek out the literature relating to research in a given subject area, only to find that the availability of this is rather limited. Although the research output is growing, the volume does not necessarily meet the needs of all practitioners for a number of reasons. The research may be plentiful in total but, when focusing on a specific subject area, there may in fact be a dearth of information. For example, when using the computerised systems now available in most professional academic libraries to identify any relevant research studies, the newcomer to research may be impressed by the volume of work undertaken and feel initially optimistic about finding work done in relation to his or her own speciality. However, if the work is very specialised he or she may find it difficult to identify any work specifically related to the subject. A good illustration of this would be to consider the rise in 'new' specialities over recent years such as the rapid growth of organ transplantation programmes. The practitioners working in this area may find research is plentiful in terms of renal and corneal transplantation, for example, but perhaps much less readily available when looking for literature on cardiac transplantation which is a more recent treatment. Alternatively there may be work available reporting on medical research in the areas interested in physiological effects of transplantation but very little in the area of psycho-social needs of patients. Traditionally it has been the pioneers of the speciality who have had the responsibility of establishing the knowledge base. However, this is another area that is changing as a result of the NHS R&D strategy as people seek to establish the benefits or otherwise of new treatment regimes. It is no longer accepted that care practice will change without some evaluation of the process. Consequently external reviews of practice are increasing.

Another aspect related to availability of research is linked to the stage of development of research for a number of health care professions. We have noted that research has been established in medical practice for a number of years and consequently this has an impact on the quantity and quality of the research produced. However, it should be noted that research in medical practice has tended to follow a very prescriptive model largely influenced by experimental approaches. As you will see later this is just one of a number of approaches to research. As nursing and other health care professionals that do not have this background in research develop their knowledge base, many reported studies are classed as 'small scale', leading to questions about the extent to which they can be utilised in practice. There is an undoubted need to replicate studies in a variety of settings to test the adequacy of the findings in a broader setting but this aspect is only developing in line with the pace of development of health care research in general. This may cause frustration for practitioners trying to find research into their area of interest. To attempt to change practice on the basis of findings from an inadequate research study could result in unsafe practices in care.

Cost of research

This subject of funding research studies will be discussed further in Chapter 4 but it has been included here to indicate that there are cost implications in preparing nurses and other health care staff to be aware of research. If we are to provide the opportunity for practitioners to study research we should consider the costs involved. Not only would teaching time need to be considered but also the costs of releasing staff from their area of practice to undertake their research studies. Costs will vary depending on the time spent in study, which can range in time from short study sessions over a few hours, to weeks or months on a more in-depth course.

Using research awareness in practice

If practitioners are to increase their research awareness they need to develop a good understanding of the research process so that they can read and understand the research that is available to them in their area of work. Only when this knowledge is available is the practitioner in a position to consider ways in which he or she can develop research awareness in his or her own clinical practice. Consequently the following chapters will consider the skills required to understand the research process. In the last chapter we will return to the issue of research awareness and expand this to consider the dissemination and utilisation of research in practice.

ACTIVITY _____

Consider, your own experiences of working within a health care team:

• Think back on your own experiences of research to date: how have you learned about this topic so far?
• How has your level of knowledge influenced your ability to use research in your work?

- List any experiences you may have of working in
    a ritualistic manner,
    an intuitive manner,
    an approach that relies on common sense.

- Identify the strengths and weaknesses of using such approaches in the context of your own examples.

Summary

The focus of this chapter has been the subject of research awareness and an attempt has been made to provide a definition for this term. Factors that may affect the level of research awareness have been discussed.

References

Benner, P. (1987) *From Novice to Expert*, Addison Wesley, Menlo Park, California.
Robinson, K. and Vaughan, B. (1992) *Knowledge for Nursing Practice*, Butterworth-Heinemann, Oxford.

Further reading

Abbott, P. and Sapsford, R. (1992) *Research Into Practice. A Reader for Nurses and the Caring Professions*, Open University Press, Buckingham.
Benner, P. (1984) *From Novice to Expert*, Addison Wesley, Menlo Park, California.
Clark, E. (1991) *Research Awareness Module 1 Nursing Research in Professional Development*, Distance Learning Centre, South Bank Polytechnic (South Bank University), London.
Reed, J. and Proctor, S. (Eds) (1995) *Practitioner Research in Health Care: The Inside Story*, Chapman & Hall, London.
Sapsford, R. and Abbott, P. (1992) *Research Methods for Nurses and the Caring Professions*, Open University Press, Buckingham.

Refer also to: The English National Board for Nursing, Midwifery and Health Visiting, 'Research Highlights' series.

3 Ideas for research

The main purpose of this chapter is to indicate how ideas for a research study may be derived. This has been included because people approaching research studies for the first time often have difficulty in determining how to focus their work. They might ask why things happen but, in following this query through, get diverted to other interesting areas of study. Alternatively they may have an interest in an area of practice but be uncertain as to where to begin planning a research study. In cases such as these, nurses and other health care workers may become diverted from an original line of enquiry and attempt to explore too many issues. Once the idea for research has been clarified the next step is to develop these into a problem statement or *research question* that will provide the basis for research. This chapter will focus on the skills required for the following:

1. To generate ideas for research.
2. To develop research questions.

Getting research ideas

The newcomer to research may be faced with a barrage of questions when thinking about research. These include issues such as where researchers get their ideas from, how they decide what specific aspects to research or how to state the research question.

These questions are just a start and, although fairly simple at first glance, it is these issues that cause a lot of anxiety to the newcomer to research. It is not uncommon for practitioners approaching research studies for the first time to feel very uncertain as to which direction to take when thinking about research ideas. They may have the ideas but be uncertain as to how to utilise them in a study of their own area of practice.

The amount of research information available through literary services is huge and unless an organised approach is taken it is very easy to get caught up in literature in such a way that the main focus of the proposed study becomes diluted. In this situation the practitioner wanting to undertake some research may become disheartened for the implications of an initial study idea may become so vast as to make any proposed project seem an impossibility. The result in this situation may be an overloading of the senses to the extent that reading stops and any further interest or development of research ideas becomes stifled. Equally, the practitioner who wants to initiate research-based practice may become so immersed in a very large area of interest that he or she is unable to instigate any changes simply because there are too many to choose from. Consequently he or she may find it difficult to be specific about which path to follow. Streamlining of ideas should help to ensure a more positive outcome in both of these situations. Consideration of how research ideas can be generated will help identify the processes that researchers go through when undertaking projects.

Research projects can be generated from two sources which can be classed as internal or external. The first, the internal source, is the individual researchers themselves who may have a specific area of interest which motivates them to develop their knowledge by undertaking research into the subject. The second, external, source is that in which the idea originates from another source such as a funding organisation, or employer which has identified an area of need for further study and consequently may employ a researcher to undertake the necessary work.

These two sources of research ideas may be closely related. For example, a practitioner working in any clinical environment may feel that some aspect of care should be closely scrutinised. She or he may then approach the employer for permission and time to undertake a research project into this area and subsequently may be given support to do this. Alternatively, the employer may recognise a need for a particular study to be done and approach a practitioner who is known to have a special interest in the topic with a request to him or her to undertake the work.

It should perhaps also be noted another 'source' of research activity relates to the occasions when another person has the original 'idea' which is then followed up by somebody else with a research interest. There are undoubtedly many 'ideas people' in our society who can inspire others to work towards achieving a goal, and the value of such people is not underestimated by researchers.

External funding bodies commission research which has been identified as a priority area. There are occasions when nurses and health care workers undertake academic courses in which a research project is part of the course requirement. If this is the case they may approach their employers for guidance on which subject areas it would be useful to research. Occasionally there are situations when employers maintain the right to choose topics for research if they are funding a member of staff through an academic course that involves a research study.

For the new researcher a good starting point for any research is to begin by looking at practice in the area in which they work. This has the advantage of making the research more meaningful and therefore perhaps helps the practitioner to maintain interest as the study becomes complex and time consuming. The major disadvantage of this approach is that in looking at practice the practitioner is faced with so many choices that it is difficult to determine exactly which aspect should be studied first.

A useful tip at this stage is to identify a 'mentor' or supervisor who will help clarify ideas. This person could help save a lot of anxiety by helping clarify ideas at an early stage in the study of research. Those people who commonly fall into the category of mentors for practitioners undertaking research are those who are seen to have some knowledge of the subject such as known researchers, teachers/lecturers or colleagues who have undertaken a research study (we will return to this topic in the next chapter).

If the newcomer to research has difficulty in clarifying research ideas he or she will need to consider how to overcome this problem. One way of doing this is to use the frameworks for care available to practitioners today.

Using a framework to generate research ideas

When trying to clarify ideas it is useful to begin with a clearly defined framework that will help structure thought processes. If this principle is applied to research in health care then it is advisable to consider what frameworks are available to guide practice. Following this line of thought one 'framework' available to nurses and other health care workers is that commonly described as the 'activities of living' (Table 3.1). Each health care professional might have a different aspect of the activities that is their prime concern, but despite this all would be alert to other activities that might impinge on the care of their client.

Table 3.1 Examples of 'activities of living' used by the health care team

- Breathing
- Eating and drinking
- Eliminating
- Personal hygiene
- Body temperature
- Mobilising
- Sleeping
- Communication
- Employment and social life

If this model was used to provide a framework to generate research ideas the researcher could, for example, create a concept map which would help identify aspects of care that could be a subject either for research or for creating a logical approach to research based on practice. This idea has been developed in Figure 3.1. Examples of activities of living have been identified and potential areas for research development drawn from this. Some of these areas can be seen to be physiological in nature, whilst others have a more psychological or sociological orientation. This is an important point to note for it reinforces the wide-ranging areas open to those wishing to undertake research in nursing and health care.

The use of this type of diagrammatic representation of research ideas is also helpful for it demonstrates how a subject area can be reduced to component parts. A newcomer to research may start off with an interest in research in which he or she states that their study will be into the area of communication in nursing. One glance at the diagram in Figure 3.1 shows that, even with just a preliminary outline, this subject is too vast to explore as a whole. The researcher needs to be much more specific in determining the focus of the study. The skill required to be specific and concise in stating the focus of a research study is one that develops with experience in research.

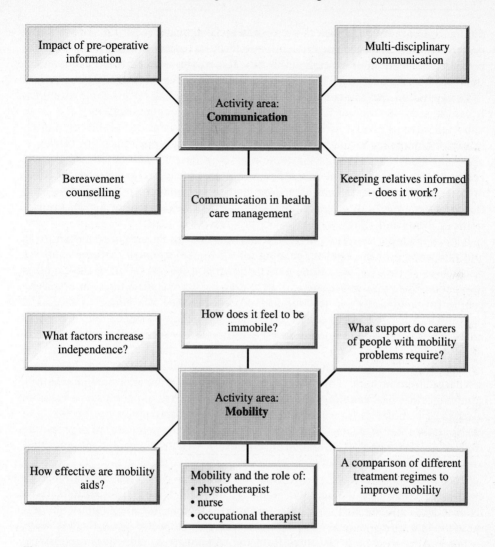

Figure 3.1 Developing areas for research from identified activities.

As you will see later it can be developed in the definition of research questions. Generally it may be noted that the more precise a researcher is in defining the boundaries of a study, the more likely he or she is to produce a valuable piece of work. The newcomer to research can quite often flounder in his or her study since lack of precision can result in lack of direction or, more commonly, may mean that the topic is too big to study properly. It should be noted that even areas identified in Figure 3.1 may be too big for a single researcher to tackle and, in reality, you might be drawing questions from the problem areas noted around the activities.

The ideas linked to each activity in Figure 3.1 are by no means conclusive and if drawn up by another writer could probably show quite a different pattern. However, the figure indicates a number of areas that could be explored from such differing perspectives as management, education or clinical practice and from different perspectives in the multi-disciplinary team. The emphasis given to any subsequent study would vary according to the specific interests of the researcher.

To expand on the points made above it may be useful to review some examples. It can be seen that one of the activity areas noted is 'communication'. This is an important area as breakdown in communication still remains one of the commonest causes of complaints in the health services today. From a research point of view it opens up many challenges as the topic may be approached from a psychological perspective in the context of counselling, from an educational perspective in terms of the impact of patient/client education, and from a managerial perspective from the points of view both of communication in the health care team and of keeping patients/clients and relatives informed of progress.

It is worth noting that a lot of research has been done in the area of communication and this work provides relevant reading for all health care staff. Awareness of the research work that has been done may help increase the utilisation of these studies in practice. The nurse in the surgical ward may have a specific interest in preparing people psychologically for the surgical procedures they are about to face. The physiotherapist may be more concerned with ensuring that this same group of patients understands the need to co-operate with post-operative exercises. In the community other members of the team may be concerned about the level of communication between themselves and hospital staff when dealing with patients who have been discharged from hospital. The manager of a unit may be more interested in exploring communication between the health care team and relatives of patients as a result of a series of complaints from patients' relatives about communication. Lecturers in health studies may be interested in communication from the point of view of preparing students in health care to communicate effectively with those people for whom they are caring.

Other aspects of research might have a stronger sociological orientation. For example in relation to the activity 'mobility', noted in Figure 3.1, questions about independence and support for carers are raised. These in turn may impact on how an individual with a mobility problem can manage in society. Again there is scope in this activity to explore the topic from the perspective of individual professional groups and from the multi-disciplinary perspective.

The ideas noted in Figure 3.1 are simply prompts towards developing research ideas. From here the next step would be to be more specific in determining your research questions.

Defining questions for research

When people approach research for the first time they find it very difficult to focus the research into a discreet area that would create a manageable research project. This is particularly so for people undertaking small-scale studies, particularly if they

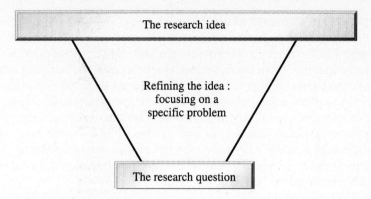

Figure 3.2 Developing the research question.

have to be completed in a limited time span. Consequently, spending time on defining the questions for research is very important as it is very easy to get side-tracked and lose the focus of the study from the outset.

Some authors have suggested that the process involved in developing a research question is rather like working your way through an inverted funnel. You start out with the broad idea of the area of study and proceed to explore only a minute part of that in the research question. This is illustrated in Figure 3.2. You can see that there is a large 'space' in the centre for refining the research idea into a research question. This is important for, as you will note throughout this text, it is the research questions that you want answered that will drive the whole research process and indicate the way in which you should approach your research.

Types of research question

Later in the text we will look at how different types of research are approached. These different types of research are required to answer specific research questions. The types of questions you might use in research can be identified at three different levels. The first level is the kind of question that asks '*What is happening here?*'. This is the sort of question you might use if you were to undertake a descriptive research study. The next level could be the kind of question that asks '*What is the relationship between the factors I am observing?*'. The research approach used for this kind of study is correlational design whilst if you ask '*How do the results from one group compare with the results from another group?*' a comparative research design is indicated. Finally you might want to ask the question '*why does this happen?*'. To ascertain the answer to that type of question you would need to be more proactive in the research design and seek to test '*cause and effect*' using experimental research design. These different research designs are discussed in more detail later in the text.

Defining the area of study

Assuming you have got to the point of deciding what type of question to ask, you need to be quite sure that you are clear in terms about the meaning attached to the terms you are using in your research to describe the *variables or particular attributes you wish to study*. Consequently you will need to develop the skills required to define concepts and propose relationships between concepts in the context of your work. This process is useful, however, in helping you to describe the main focus of your study and from this, the other aspect might be considered as subsidiary to your idea. The process might inform the way in which you will collect data for research. We will return to this later in Chapter 6.

ACTIVITY _____

Think about your own area of practice:

- Make a list of broad aspects of care that are relevant to your own professional role (use the activities of living framework if appropriate).
- From this identify an aspect of care that you may like to research.
- In diagrammatic form (as in Figure 3.1) indicate a range of questions that you could ask related to your chosen aspect of care.
- Choose one area only and write a research question you would like to answer (we will return to this later in the text).

Summary

This chapter has outlined some areas from which research ideas could be generated and research questions developed. The use of a framework to structure thinking when developing research ideas has been recommended.

Further reading

Berger, R.M. and Patchup, M.A. (1988) *Planning for Research, A Guide for the Helping Professions*, Sage, London.
Brink, P.J. and Wood, M.J. (1988) *Basic Steps in Planning Nursing Research*, Jones & Bartlett, Boston.
Brockopp, D.Y. and Hastings-Tolsma, M.T. (1995) *Fundamentals of Nursing Research*, 2nd edn, Jones & Bartlett, Boston.
Clarke, E. (1991) *Research Awareness Module 5 Identifying and Refining Research Questions*, Distance Learning Centre, South Bank Polytechnic (South Bank University), London.
Clifford, C., Carnwell, R. and Harkin, L. (1996) *Research Methodology in Nursing and Health Care*, Open Learning Foundation/Churchill Livingstone, Edinburgh.
Cormack, D.F.S. (1991) *The Research Process in Nursing*, 2nd edn, Blackwell Scientific Publications, Oxford.

Polit, D.F. and Hunglar, B.P. (1992) *Nursing Research, Principles and Methods*, J.B. Lipincot and Company, Philadelphia.

Roper, N., Logan, W.W. and Tierney, A. (1996) *The Elements of Nursing. A Model for Nursing Based on a Model for Living*, 4th edn, Churchill Livingstone, Edinburgh.

4   Planning for research

Research projects of any sort do put big demands on the researcher and the nature of research often means that there may be times when plans do not develop as desired. All newcomers to research should be aware of the factors that might impinge on research so that they use time and energy well throughout the study and recognise that there will be times of despondency as well as times of satisfaction when all appears to be going to plan. This chapter outlines some of the practical issues that should be considered when planning a research project and considers the following:

1. Supervisor/mentor support.
2. Research experience.
3. Planning time.
4. Funding research.
5. Ethical issues.
6. Access.

The importance of planning cannot be underestimated in any research project and skills in project planning need to be nurtured from an early stage when people are interested in undertaking research. Careful planning at all stages will not only help towards achieving a better quality research study but, more importantly from the researcher's point of view, it will also save a lot of time and effort as the study progresses. For example, when decorating a room, colour schemes are planned and the surfaces carefully prepared for a new coat of paint. The benefits of this are obvious to any experienced decorator. The results of careful planning and preparation are that in anticipating what needs to be done in the early stages, delays are avoided, all the necessary equipment is at hand and the quality of the end result reflects the planning and preparation. So it is with the researcher: careful consideration of all of the issues involved and a plan that is well structured and logical in relation to all aspects of the research process can help avoid problems as the study is developed and can enhance the quality of the completed work.

   In the previous chapter the challenges faced by a researcher trying to work up new ideas for research, deciding the problem area and defining the research question were considered. Obviously this must be the starting point for any research project. Unless you are clear about the area of interest for your research you will be starting to plan from a very shaky foundation. Being clear about the area of interest does not mean, at the outset, that you have to have every aspect of the research covered; it simply means that you need to be sure of the focus of your work so that you do not go off in all directions and lose that focus. This is important when it comes to making maximum use of the time available to you for any research-related activity.

Supervisor/mentor support

Experienced researchers will know the value of having a research supervisor to advise and guide their progress through more complex studies. A supervisor will offer support and advice to a researcher undertaking a project and, more importantly, they may help save time by helping avoid those errors that frustrate researchers in moments of crisis throughout any research project. As noted in Chapter 3 it is advisable to identify a mentor or supervisor from the outset when clarifying areas for research as advice at this point can help avoid a lot of frustration in the early stages of a study.

Health care practitioners undertaking research as part of an academic course of study will usually have a supervisor identified as they begin their work. However, staff working in clinical areas and wishing to undertake research may need to look around to identify a suitable person for this role. This may be a colleague who has had some experience of doing research themselves or a more senior member of staff who feels able to guide and give support and advice when required. If there is no-one in the immediate work environment to give support of this nature then a review of personnel working in the locality might identify people who may be able to act in a supervisory capacity. For example, there may be someone working in a local R&D unit or someone working in a local university who could help.

In addition there may be an active research interest group available locally. Members of such groups are generally supportive towards each other when developing research projects and so may be helpful in identifying resources.

Research experience

The experience of the researcher is another factor that will influence the planning of research and deciding what supervision support is required. Newcomers to research may be advised to start with a simple project first. Many experienced researchers can identify the difficulties they encountered in undertaking their first research studies and will note the value of learning the pitfalls of research before getting involved in a major project. The research process is not one of those things that can be learned from reading textbooks, it is a process that is best learned by doing. In 'doing' research a lot of insight can be gained that cannot be gathered from a book, however widely read the individual.

In doing a small-scale study researchers may not be able to generalise the findings to a variety of settings, but this does not mean that the work will have no value. As you will see in Chapter 6 small-scale research projects may not provide a sound base for major developments in care but, in contributing to the total body of knowledge in a given topic, they may add to the knowledge base which eventually provides a base for the developing practice. If a number of small-scale studies are replicated and the same results identified, ultimately it may be possible to generalise findings based on cumulative evidence. Moreover, newcomers to research need to learn about the process of research and small-scale projects help new researchers recognise the potential pitfalls of completing research.

Planning time

A skill that is an essential prerequisite to developing a good research project is time management. Health care workers who undertake research for the first time often do not appreciate how time consuming it is to carry out a well-planned research project. As a result they can get very frustrated with the work while it is in progress simply because of pressures on time. Consequently the researcher needs to consider how much time is available to him or her to undertake their project. This will effectively set the boundaries for the study you might want to undertake.

For example, if a physiotherapist was on a part time degree programme which required that during the course of the last year a small-scale research project must be undertaken, he or she might look at the diary and realise that the time available to undertake the project work was limited to half a day per week for a twelve week period. If, for the project, the physiotherapist wanted to explore aspects of rehabilitation following a stroke it may rapidly become apparent that the size of any such project will be limited to a small number of patients or clients attending his or her own clinical area. In contrast, if the physiotherapist had been awarded a research scholarship that allowed time for a full time research project over three years then the boundaries of the study will be far greater.

In both instances the physiotherapist has the same area of interest but the person working part time would not be able to carry out the same in-depth project as the full time researcher. Consequently although both might have started with the same idea, such as 'What is the impact of physiotherapy following a stroke?', the limitations imposed on the part time research may be such that the physiotherapist can only ask the question 'What are patients' perception of physiotherapy following a stroke?'. It is not uncommon for researchers to modify their initial ideas in this way to come up with a research study that is feasible in the time available. The ideal is to look for ways to find time to undertake research studies and it is from this perspective that we will look at funding for research. To help in time management researchers will often be advised to design a time plan to indicate defined research activities over the period of time allocated to the study.

Funding research

In this section funding for research will be considered from several perspectives. The first is the sources of funding available to health care workers, and the second is the way in which you might calculate the costs of a given project. The skills required in relation to funding issues in research include being alert to the ways in which sources of funding are identified and some simple skill in developing costing models for research projects. Finally, assuming that funds were awarded, managing the funds allocated to the project is a skill in its own right. Each of these will be considered below.

Sources of funding

Although quite a lot of small-scale research is carried out without application for funds, some source of funding may be necessary to undertake more complex studies. The amount of financial support sought through funding agencies can vary from small sums that will help offset the costs of producing research instruments, through to full funding which includes paying salaries for the researcher and assistants in addition to all other anticipated expenditure.

The sources of funding for research are varied and can range from the employer through to national bodies in both professional and voluntary capacities. This includes professional organisations, research councils (such as the Medical Research Council), Department of Health, NHS R&D strategic development programme and major charities. The potential researcher has to be alert to the availability of such funds. The increased awareness of funding sources is a skill that potential researchers can develop. Broadly speaking the main sources of information about the availability of research funds are as follows:

1. Libraries that stock directories of charitable organisations that may be approached with applications for research funds. This includes public libraries and academic libraries depending on the area of interest.
2. Newspapers and professional journals advertise funds awarded from the major charities and through the NHS R&D strategy.
3. Professional organisations, again commonly advertising these through professional journals.
4. Advice from colleagues or managers who have experience of seeking funds for research or colleagues working in the university sector who may have developed their own data base of funding sources.
5. Increasingly computer networks are becoming a source of information using the Internet/e-mail.

The demand for funds for research exceeds the resources available and so the researcher may need to spend a lot of time and energy in the search for funding. Indeed most researchers will tell you that this can be a very disheartening experience as the search for funding from research is becoming more and more competitive. The skills required to apply for funds in the first instance are the skills necessary to plan a research study and write a research proposal. This will be examined in some depth in Chapter 11. One component of preparing a research proposal is how to calculate the costs of funding research and this will be considered below.

Calculating the costs of research projects

The financial implications of research should always be considered at an early stage of planning for research. This is an important lesson for the beginner since if a researcher at this stage can learn the cost implications of investing time and resources into a small-scale project the lessons learned can be transferred to more substantive projects at a later stage if appropriate.

The focus in this section will be to show you how to work out the costs for a project yourself. The same principles apply for funding for a relatively small-scale project that would be undertaken part time as for more extensive funds to support a full time research project. However, whilst you might be expected to produce your own funding outline for relatively small sums of money you can be reassured that if you were in a position to apply for more substantive funds, the funding organisation would expect that you have support from the financial managers in the organisation in which your research project will be located. Consequently you may be in a position to seek professional advice from an accountant when developing this. Even so, it is still important that you understand the principles of funding research and these are outlined below.

There are two broad categories that should be considered when costing a research project: personnel costs and the other resources required to support the project, as indicated in Table 4.1.

Table 4.1 Broad categories for costing a research project

Personnel
Researcher time
Secretarial support
Any other specialist advice required, e.g. supervisor time, statistical advice
On costs

Other resources
Stationary and photocopying
Postage
Travel
Computing facilities
Any other, e.g. contingency

Personnel

By far the biggest cost to any research project is the *time* required by the *researcher* to undertake the project work. Most health care workers are not used to considering the cost implications for their time, for unless they are working regularly in agencies which offer an hourly rate it is not something that occurs to them. Consequently when it comes to costing research it is easy to underestimate the cost implications of researcher time.

The way in which you would cost your 'research time' if you wanted to undertake a project is to find out the hourly rate for the job you do and then calculate the number of hours, over the specified number of weeks or months, that you anticipate the research project will take. So for example, if an occupational therapist wanted to undertake a project designed to assess the capability levels of people being discharged from hospital following a stroke, he or she may plan a small-scale research project that is anticipated to take twelve weeks to complete. If each working week is 37 hours this gives a total of 444 hours. He or she may check with the finance department what their 'hourly rate' of pay is; let us say this is £15 per hour for our example. The therapist now has the data to undertake the first step of the costing exercise. To calculate how much his or her time will cost therefore, the occupational therapist needs to multiply the total number of hours by the cost per hour as illustrated in Table 4.2. This shows the total cost for the time required by the occupational therapist to complete this research project is £6660.

Table 4.2 Calculating the cost of time spent on research project

Number of weeks for project (12) × Number of hours per week (37) = 444 hours
Total number of hours (444) × Rate per hour (£15)   = £6660

You should also consider any requirements you might have for *secretarial* help. With the advent of word processors many people undertaking research find that they can do their own typing and again may perceive this as being a 'saving' when costing a project. However, there are again some cost implications here. If, for example, the occupational therapist above was costing his or her time for this project at £15 per hour and included within that was time for typing questionnaires and reports, this may not be a good use of resources. The costs of secretarial time vary depending on the level of skill required but generally the occupational therapist may expect a higher rate of pay than a secretary, given current rates of pay. Consequently if, for example, it was noted that we could get an experienced secretary to work on our project at a rate of £7.50 per hour it is more cost effective for a secretary to do the typing associated with the project than it is for the researcher. The cost per hour for a secretary is half that of the occupational therapist. In a small-scale study such as our example referred to here we might need a limited amount of secretarial time, let us say two weeks' worth of activity (2 weeks × 37 hours per week = 74 hours in total). This will give us a total cost of £555 as illustrated in Table 4.3.

Table 4.3 Calculating the cost of secretarial time spent on research project

Number of weeks for project (2) × Number of hours per week (37) = 74 hours
Total number of hours (74) × Rate per hour (£7.50)   = £555

The same formula is used to cost the time required by *other personnel* involved in the project include the potential for involving research *supervisor* time in the funding although the need for this will vary. For example if you are undertaking a research project as part of a formal course of study in a local university you do not need to consider this as it will already be costed in your fees for the course you are doing.

However, if you were applying for funds to enable you to undertake a project in clinical areas you might need to consider who you can approach to help you in this. Depending on the size, the nature of the project and the locality of the potential supervisor you might need to consider allowing funds to support you. For example if you had a colleague who was an experienced researcher who could provide the kind of supervision for mentorship advice you needed for your project you might find they were willing to help you but had to account for time to their manager. Consequently you might need to make an allowance for that for costing purposes. In our example £1000 is allowed for supervisor time which may include 20–30 hours (at a rate of £30–£50 per hour) of time spent by the supervisor working with you on the project, guiding and directing your activities, helping you with collecting information or reading your reports (see Table 4.4).

Table 4.4 Example of costing for a research project over a three month period

Personnel	
Researcher time	£6660
Secretarial support	£555
Any other specialist advice required	
Supervisor	£1000
Statistical advice	£500
On costs on salary (at 10%)	
Researcher	£666
Secretary	£555
Other resources	
Stationary (1 pack of paper)	£10
Photocopying (600 sides at 10p)	£60
Postage (25p × 2 for each 100 respondents)	£50
(Travel – not required)	
Computing facilities (not required)	
Any other	
Contingency	£200
Total	**£10256**

Any other specialist advice required is determined by the specific requirements of each project but, generally speaking, this may include help with *statistical analysis* if undertaking a study that involved this type of testing. It is worth noting that many universities and other 'specialist' services such as those provided by statisticians are well used to costing their time and commonly work to a fixed formula decided by the organisation concerned. Consequently if you were to seek this kind of specialist advice you might expect that the experts themselves will be able to cost this quite quickly for you. We have allowed £500 for this, which might give 10–15 hours (allowing £30–£50 per hour) of time spent by a statistician helping you to analyse your data.

For simplicity the number of personnel involved in the example has been kept to a minimum. Increasingly the pattern in health care is to develop research studies that involve a team of researchers looking at a specific research problem from differing angles and so it might be that this section in a costing bid could contain, at a minimum, time for a single researcher, and at a maximum, a research team consisting of several members of the health care team.

On costs

The last item listed in Table 4.1 under the heading of personnel is what is called 'on costs'. This is a concept that is familiar to financial managers but not one which most of us have cause to consider. Basically 'on costs' refer to the additional costs an employer meets in employing us. It is a levy that is applied to all employees' salaries to cover employers' contributions to national insurance and so on. When calculating research costs we need to add the on costs to the basic salary to give the real cost of research time. For example, if the occupational therapist undertaking this project wanted to get sufficient funds to enable him or her to undertake this project for three months we have noted that, taking the hourly rate, this can be costed at £6660. The 'on costs' for an employee can vary from 10 to 15 per cent; for simplicity let us assume that in this case it is 10 per cent, which of £6660 is £666. So the real cost of our occupational therapist taking time out to do this project is £7326 (i.e. £6660 + £666). Thus you can see estimating the real cost (basic salary plus on cost) can make quite a difference to the overall total.

At this stage of thinking about research you might ask yourself why we are bothering with the 'on costs' or 'Why don't the managers support this?'. The simple answer is that we live and work in a world where money is an important consideration. If the occupational therapist wants to take time out of work to do this project then his or her manager has to be able to replace his or her time in the service structure so that the work can be done. If the 'on costs' were not considered in the research funding the managers would in effect be subsidising the time out to the tune of £666 and they would also have to pay the full cost for the replacement therapist.

Other resources

As with the number of personnel so the range of resources required to support individual studies will vary. Several things have been listed, including *stationary*, *photocopying* and *postage costs*. Again these can be severely underestimated by the researcher. Newcomers to research commonly say that their study will not cost much for they are doing it in their 'own time' and are only, for example, going to circulate a questionnaire. Let us consider the example of a questionnaire that will be circulated to 100 people. If each questionnaire consists of four sides of A4 paper that totals 200 sheets of paper and 400 pages of copying. Your own local stationary suppliers will help you cost this but if, for example, each page of photocopying cost 10 pence then copying 400 sheets would total £40. That is of course just for the finished product. It is likely that you will print many more copies when developing the questionnaire and testing it.

You then need to add to this the cost of paper, envelopes to post the questionnaire to respondents, envelopes for the return of the questionnaires from respondents, and any postage costs this incurs if relevant.

Depending on the way you collect information you may need to consider *telephone charges* or *travel expenses*, although travel costs may not be a consideration if using questionnaires. However, if instead of this approach to collecting information, the research was going to necessitate interviewing people or completing some observation, you will need to include costs for this as, again, this soon mounts up over a period of time.

The cost for *computing facilities* will depend on the availability of local resources, but if the researcher does not have access to these they must be costed out also.

The 'any other' category is a useful category for considering other costs that might arise out of the research. For example the researcher may be asked to participate in conferences to talk about the project, or might find in the middle of the project that some interesting line of enquiry develops. Consequently it is useful in any research project to have a little *contingency* fund for this, for example, to help with disseminating research (see Chapter 12). It is not uncommon now for researchers to include a cost for dissemination in a bid for funds. For the sake of our example we will include a contingency of £200 for this small-scale project, although in some larger studies this would be a bigger sum.

University or institutional on costs

One further aspect not considered is that of the costs involved in providing office space, lighting, etc., to the researcher. Whilst this is not perhaps so relevant to small-scale projects such as in the example in Table 4.4, it is an important consideration if you are ever involved in completing the costing for major projects. For example if a research funding bid included the costs of two researchers over a one or two year period, both would require office space. It is because of the costs incurred in providing office facilities that universities and other institutions often levy an additional 'on cost' for use of such resources. This cost will vary, depending on the institution but generally speaking it is between 25 and 40 per cent of the total costs of personnel involved in the project. You will see this additional cost 'in action' if you are ever involved in putting in a bid for research funds with university staff.

So in summary, even at a basic level researchers need to consider that time costs money. An illustration of how this costing might look in a bid for research funds can be seen in Table 4.4. This will also serve to illustrate to you the potential cost impact of a health care professional undertaking a research project, for our total sum is calculated at £10,256 yet, at the beginning of this section, it was noted this would be a 'small-scale' project. Even if a practitioner is undertaking a small research project in his or her own unit, there is an initial cost implication based on the time allocated for undertaking the research and the basic resources required to complete that work. This point is not made to discourage research being undertaken during working hours but rather to emphasise that no research project is free of financial consideration.

Finally, on the issue of costing a project, it is also important to consider the cost in relation to the time spent by respondents when participating in the study. Admittedly this may be a 'hidden' cost but researchers need to be aware of this when planning research projects, for this may affect the willingness of people to participate in the study. For example, if members of the multi-disciplinary health care team allocated to one clinical unit were asked to participate in an interview lasting one hour the time involved could be extensive and may affect willingness to participate in the project.

Managing funds awarded for research

In this introductory text it is not appropriate to spend a lot of time considering how to manage research funds. However, it is important to point out that if as a health care worker you were awarded a research grant through the major sources of funding for research, this would be administered through the finance department in your place of employment. Consequently the way in which you would access the funds will be directed by the system in operation in your own locality. Thus the management of any research grant requires the support of the financial managers in your organisation. This is quite reassuring for those researchers who have not had experience in managing project funds although, when first faced with setting up a system for managing funds, it can be quite an unnerving experience. Most funding agencies recognise that the management issues can be complex and often scrutinise the members of a *research team* on larger projects to identify whether there is this kind of experience.

Ethical issues

One of the major difficulties facing researchers is determining when it is acceptable to continue with the study in hand and when it should be discontinued because the work transcends the boundaries of what may be considered acceptable from an ethical point of view. A research supervisor should be in a position to give an objective view on this aspect of any proposed study. Indeed one of the benefits of having a good supervisor is that he or she would not let you proceed with any study that was likely to have any major ethical implications or cause undue suffering to anyone participating in the research.

As knowledge of research in health care increases, practitioners are becoming more skilled at determining which areas of study may engender ethical dilemmas. However, along with this increasing knowledge of ethics in research comes increasing knowledge in health care with the rapid advances in technological development. This can cause major concerns to those responsible for determining whether a study should be allowed to proceed on ethical grounds. For example new drugs for treating cancer are constantly being developed. To determine whether such drugs work they do need to be tested on real patients with real problems. Is it ethically acceptable to approach people for whom no other line of treatment is available and ask them to participate in a research study that may involve additional discomfort as a result of the drugs?

Another example might be a situation when a nurse wants to study the stress that a diagnosis of cancer may bring to his or her patients. The rationale for this is that if he or she understands better how the patients feel, he or she may be able to provide better care. Given that the patients may have only just been told of the diagnosis, they are bound to be very distressed. To ask such a person to participate in a research study at this time may create additional suffering. To add to the distress of the individual would be in conflict with good ethical principles for that individual yet the knowledge gained is aimed at alleviating suffering wherever possible. Obviously each of these examples needs to be considered carefully and consequently the format of any proposed research should be critically and sensitively planned to ensure that no additional suffering occurs.

The way in which it is proposed the study is to be carried out is relevant to these ethical dilemmas. For example, distress may occur if an approach is adopted in which the researcher goes, with a clipboard in hand, and briskly asks the patient direct questions from a structured questionnaire about the 'stress' they are experiencing. The nature of the subject under review lends itself to a more subtle approach in determining the patient's reactions to the condition. Informal interviews are an alternative that may be utilised, for conversational techniques may be less stressful than the rigid format of a structured interview using a questionnaire.

The timing of the study is another consideration. Although the researcher may want to identify the initial reaction of the patient it may be better to undertake this work at a later date. This means that the information is gathered after the event and the data are based on recall rather than the 'here and now'. This technique of gathering data *retrospectively* is quite commonly used in research. It can be contrasted with a *prospective* approach in which the researcher anticipates collecting data in the future.

Although the approaches outlined above reflect differences in research methodology, what is at issue here is not the research method, but the effect that different approaches to research may have on the individual being studied. It is essential that the researcher considers all of these factors from an ethical point of view when planning research projects.

Ethical committees

It is recognised that there are occasions when researchers, in their pursuit of knowledge, may face ethical dilemmas when determining the boundaries of their study. To ensure that the interests and safety of the public are maintained it is important that an external agency monitors the work of researchers.

Ethical committees are a well-established means of doing this in health care. The purpose of these committees is to ensure that any research undertaken, involving members of the general public in particular, is not of itself likely to cause any degree of distress or harm to those individuals participating in the study. In terms of planning for research it is important that the potential researcher finds out two things:

1. How the ethical committees work in their own health district.
2. What the ethical committee needs to know.

How the ethical committees work

In the context of the first point, how ethical committees work, gaining ethical approval can be quite a time-consuming process as the frequency with which such committees meet is varied. If, for example the committee meets monthly and for some reason it has queries about your application for ethical approval of a proposed research study it might be a couple of months before you get approval to proceed. Consequently this is not something that should be left to the last minute; rather you should seek ethical approval at the earliest possible stage in planning your research. Indeed it is worth noting that a number of organisations that fund research in health care will not review applications until ethical approval has been given.

Because of local variations it is essential that health care workers wishing to undertake research clarify the approvals system within their own health district before embarking on any research study.

What the ethical committee needs to know

In Chapter 11 the factors you need to consider when preparing a plan for your research or, as commonly described, *a research proposal*, will be considered. Broadly speaking the information you present to an ethical committee will reflect the format of a research proposal. The ethical committee will need to know what you are going to do in your research, how you are going to do it, to whom you are going to do it, how you will analyse your data and what you will do with the findings from the research. In other words they will need to have a clear picture of how your research will develop. To help you in this, most ethical committees will produce a form which they ask you to complete, outlining your proposed research study. As with all official organisations you should note that if the committee ask you to complete its form you should do so. This can appear quite cumbersome at first, but generally the headings in such forms are the same as those discussed in Chapter 11 in the context of preparing research proposals.

The potential ethical dilemmas faced by ethical committees in health care can be wide and varied but, given that most researchers will have thought through the ethical issues quite carefully before commencing with the research, it is not unreasonable to suggest that the commonest problems for health workers lie in the areas of access to information and informed consent.

Access to information

This is related to the right of individuals to privacy in terms of information that is made publicly available to them. Several years ago in the United Kingdom the Data Protection Act was introduced by government to protect those individual rights to privacy. It has important implications for researchers both from the point of view of collecting information and in writing information in research reports. The details of the act are complex and beyond the scope of this book to explore but the principles can be broadly outlined in terms of health care research and ownership of data.

We all have the right to know what is written about us in any public medium. If people contact us and ask us to participate in a research study into health care because they know we have recently used the service then we have the right to know how they 'know' that. If this researcher was a member of staff at the hospital or community unit we might realise that the data have been drawn from hospital records by 'authorised' personnel. However, if this letter came from a student on a health studies degree programme we might rightly ask 'how do they know I was in hospital?'. The important point here is that a student on a health studies programme does not have the right of access to records of health care without asking for permission first. This applies even if the student is a qualified practitioner working as a professional in an NHS trust. Rights of access to details about a patient as part of care giving is not the same as rights of access for research purposes. The student may overcome this problem by asking the hospital manager or some other authority figure to circulate the letter so the student does not contact the participant directly.

Informed consent

The next issue is to ensure that people who might participate in the research are fully informed that they have a choice as to whether or not to participate in a study and that they know what will be expected of them if they do participate. To this end a major area of interest to members of ethical committees is how this information will be given to patients/clients or members of the general public participating in research studies and they usually expect that this will be in the form of some kind of written information.

Depending on the nature of the study a letter of introduction from the researcher may be sufficient. The amount of detail you put in this will depend on the nature of the study. Any covering letter should cover some key points, including who you are, what you want to do and why. You should also take opportunity to note that any participation is entirely voluntary and, particularly in the case of health care practitioners asking patients/clients to participate, it is important to ensure that potential participants do not feel that a wish not to participate will result in any change in treatment. The confidential nature of any data collected should also be stressed. Generally speaking, a well-written letter will give sufficient information for a research study that is not considered very invasive, for example if respondents are being asked to complete a questionnaire. It should be noted that any letters sent from participants should be sent from an 'official address', whether that be your place of work if appropriate or the university in which you are studying if you are a student. This is important both for verifying your authenticity to the participant and to protect your own privacy. If you are completing a research study as part of a university programme you may find it is local policy for your supervisor to countersign any letters sent to participants. This ensures that the supervisor is aware of actions that you are taking and would be able to advise you of the best approach to take when contacting clients (see Table 4.5).

Table 4.5 Example of information letter to potential research participants

[Insert work/university address]

Dear ....

I am a physiotherapist working in .... unit. I am studying for a degree of health studies and as part of my work I going to undertake a research study exploring clients' attitudes to .... I hope this work will be useful in helping us to improve our service to clients in this unit.

I am writing to you to ask if you would be able to help with this work by completing the questionnaire attached. The questionnaires are anonymous and, although I will be writing a report of my research, any names or locations of the research will not be identified in that report. All information you give will therefore be in absolute confidence.

Your help with this study is entirely voluntary and if you would prefer not to take part your care/treatment will not be affected in any way.

This study is supported by Ms .... who is the director of this unit and is supervising my research. If you would like any further information before deciding about this work please contact me or Ms .... on .... [insert Tel. no.].

If you do complete the questionnaire please return it to me in the stamped addressed envelope attached by [insert date]. If you prefer not to do so thank you for taking the time to read this letter.

Yours sincerely

.... (Physiotherapist)

.... (Research Supervisor)

As noted above a letter may give sufficient information if the research is not considered to be invasive. However, if the research demands more of the participants it may be necessary to give more information. This would apply particularly if the study demanded any change in treatment regimes. Many ethics committees recommend a fairly standardised approach to this as, if a standard 'formula' is followed, it is easier to ensure that potential research subjects receive all the appropriate information required. The key points that would be considered in an information leaflet telling potential research subjects about their research are listed in Table 4.6. The important point when preparing such information leaflets is to ensure that it is written in a style that is accessible to the person who will be reading it. It is not uncommon for newcomers to research to write the information sheet for potential respondents in quite a 'jargonistic' style. You need to avoid medical terms and write any such information sheets in 'lay terms' so that people can understand what is required of them.

Detailed information sheets such as this are commonly accompanied by a consent form which participants sign to indicate they would be willing to participate in the study. In health care research copies of the signed consent are filed in the patients'/clients' medical records.

Table 4.6 Example of headings that may be used in information sheets for potential respondents about a research study

Heading: **Title of the study**

- What is the study about?
- What will I be expected to do?
- Are there any benefits?
- Are there any risks?
- How long will the study last?
- How much of my time is required?
- What are the alternatives?
- What happens with the information? – how will I know it is confidential?
- Who else is taking part?
- What happens if I don't want to take part?
- What if something goes wrong?
- What happens at the end of the study?
- What happens if I have more questions or don't understand something?

Access

Permission for access to undertake research differs from ethical permission in that it is the responsibility of managers to determine whether it is acceptable or appropriate for a particular research project to be carried out in a given clinical area. In so doing managers will want to know whether the research has, or will have, the approval of an ethical committee but they will also be concerned about the local issues such as the impact on resources, or whether certain groups of patients in the health care trust are being over-exposed to research.

The formality involved in seeking permission for access to undertake research may vary. It may be sufficient for the manager to state that it is acceptable for the research study to proceed as long as those people directly involved are approached and permission for participation obtained directly from them.

For example a nurse may wish to study methods of work in his or her own unit as part of his or her own learning of the research process. The permission of the ward or unit manager may be all that is required to do this. If the nurse manager feels that the implications of such a study extend beyond that ward or unit he or she may then advise the potential researcher to seek permission to undertake their research through more formal channels.

It is important to stress that there are many local variations in this so any practitioner intending to do research should clarify the local procedures for seeking permission before proceeding with the study. From an ethical, and purely courteous, perspective no one should undertake a research project without discussing it first with the managers concerned.

There will be occasions when the researcher does not wish to liaise directly with the immediate manager in the unit to be studied for fear of introducing bias into the study. For example if the researcher wished to monitor ways in which work was organised in a unit it is possible that the approach to work might change as a result

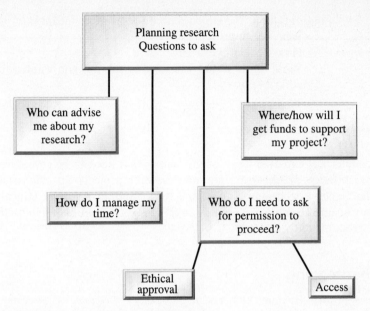

Figure 4.1 Planning research – questions to ask at the outset.

of his or her observations if staff knew they were being monitored. (The reasons for this are discussed in Chapter 9.) Consequently each case has to be considered in detail and the level at which permission for the research is sought from management should match the requirements for the study.

Another aspect related to management is that of gaining the co-operation of all those other people who may be directly or indirectly involved with the research. Many projects have succeeded only because co-operation was willingly given; the acknowledgements printed in most research papers serve to reinforce this point. Co-operation from all participants is like a tonic to the researcher, lack of support at times of need can result in despondency and frustration.

To recap before you begin your research project it is useful to consider these background issues, summarised in Figure 4.1, to avoid complications as the work progresses.

ACTIVITY _____

- Consider your own working environment and identify whether there is anyone who could act in the position of research supervisor or mentor to you.
- Imagine you were going to undertake a small study that would take twenty days of your time and involved posting questionnaires to 150 people. Calculate how much you think this would cost.

- Find out about the ethics committees in your locality:
    Who organises them?
    How frequently do they meet?
    What forms would you need to fill in if you wanted to apply for ethical approval?

Summary

This chapter has explored some of the factors that need to be considered by health care practitioners planning to undertake research projects. Specific issues addressed included supervisor support, managing time, funding research, ethical issues and access. Consideration of these wide-ranging issues should help avoid complications as the research study develops.

Further reading

Berger, R.M. and Patchup, M.A. (1988) *Planning for Research, A Guide for the Helping Professions*, Sage, London.

Cormack, D.F.S. (1991) *The Research Process in Nursing*, 2nd edn, Blackwell Scientific, Oxford.

Clifford, C., Carnwell, R. and Harkin, L. (1996) *Research Methodology in Nursing and Health Care*, Open Learning Foundation/Churchill Livingstone, Edinburgh.

Evans, D. and Evans, M. (1996) *A Decent Proposal: Ethical Review of Clinical Research*, Wiley, Chichester.

Locke, L.F., Spirduso, W.W. and Siverman, S.J. (1993) *Proposals that Work: A Guide for Planning Dissertations and Grant Proposals*, Sage, London.

See also: 'Ethical Issues and Research', *Nurse Researcher*, vol. 3, no. 1, September (1995).

5   Considering the approach to research

In this chapter we will consider some of the issues that underpin the way in which research is developed. This is important because the newcomer to research in health care is faced with a range of approaches to research that can be baffling and confusing at the outset as apparently contrary perspectives are offered as the 'right way' in which research should be developed. Consequently this includes a review of the following:

1. The philosophical basis of research.
2. The way in which knowledge is developed.
3. Developing knowledge through different approaches to research.

The impact of these issues can be seen in the overall approach to research. For example reports of research studies completed in health care might give accounts of how a small number of patients feel about their illness, an approach that can be contrasted with studies of large numbers of patients participating in studies of new drugs designed to determine the effectiveness of a new drug. Broadly speaking these approaches can be broken down into considering how we might research what people think and feel about the world around us, commonly categorised under the heading of *qualitative* research, compared with things that we can observe in a more objective way, such as the physiological response to a new drug in a large group of patients. Research which leads to development of some kind of measures of observations on larger groups of people can be described as *quantitative* research. We will return to these categories in more detail later in the chapter.

Both qualitative and quantitative approaches to research have their place in health practice yet, on occasion, the differing approaches appear as conflicting rather than complementary philosophies of research in health care. To understand why this is we need to consider the underlying philosophy of research and how this may influence health care.

The philosophical basis of research

The purpose of research is to generate knowledge but definitions of what constitutes knowledge have served to challenge philosophers over many years. Whilst to 'know' something implies that one may feel certain of the 'truth' or accuracy of a given situation, dictionary definitions of knowledge may refer more broadly to familiarity with facts, or feelings or experiences of an individual or groups. It could be suggested that it is the distinction between knowledge of facts and knowledge of feelings and experiences that provides a distinction between different approaches to research and the underlying philosophical basis of research.

Knowledge of 'facts' from the perspective of what may be considered 'true or false' in a given situation has traditionally been associated with knowledge generated through research in which care is taken to separate out the 'facts' from the 'assumptions' associated with feelings or personal experiences about a given situation. However, this is not always a straightforward process. To claim that research is about helping us to discern facts from assumptions presupposes that in all situations everything can be broken down into factual units. Unfortunately, or fortunately perhaps, when dealing with people this is not so easy; life is not like that. Whilst we may be able to categorise some human behaviours and responses (such as physiological response) into factual units it is not so easy to do this, for example, when we try to analyse human feelings or emotions.

Knowledge development: philosophical reasoning

There are some aspects of knowledge that have been developed by a process of logical reasoning and make no claim to 'factual' status from the perspective of being true or false. For example, philosophers who reason about the purpose of life have little in the way of substantive factual knowledge to support them, yet many support the logic behind differing perspectives or ways of viewing the world. Such insights enhance the humanity of our existence and encourage us to challenge, question and explore the world around us. Whether or not people are in agreement with the outcome of a particular philosophical school of thought is not always the issue – rather it is about challenging the thought processes behind the thinking and looking for flaws in the argument posed that contribute towards understanding humanity. Overall we can conclude that in philosophical reasoning knowledge is developed at an *abstract* level as there may be very little in the way of observable facts to support ideas proposed.

There are few that would question the impact of the great philosophers in developing ways of viewing the world. However, it should be noted that such views of the world are influenced by 'space and time'; in other words, where you are in the world and at what historical time will serve to influence your thinking. For example, if you were born in the late 1800s in the United Kingdom the pervading religious influences would have been Christianity: you would not have thought it likely that within a hundred years people would widely accept different religious viewpoints and ways of worship in this country. Likewise the major forms of transport would have been by foot or by horse-drawn carriage. In the 1800s you would have been very amused if you had been presented with the notion of flying over the world in aeroplanes, not to mention the thought of man landing on the moon.

In recognising how our own life experiences influence the way in which we develop our knowledge base you have only to reflect on the way you learned about life. Your early experiences for example may have convinced you that there was a 'Father Christmas' – this would have been supported by the 'evidence' of presents arriving at Christmas and to some extent your own observation of 'Father Christmas' in the local grotto. If you were in a position to visit children in other parts of the world you would have found that many of them had never heard of Father Christmas – it is only your experiences that led you to believe in this. In reality your experiences in this case would have proved false as the presents were not left by Father Christmas and the image you saw in the grotto was only a representation of an idea.

Similarly you can identify a range of culturally determined beliefs that have arisen from different experiences; for example, the perceived power of the witch doctor, or the fear that still may be exhibited in response to an eclipse of the sun in some cultures and so on. In these situations people are simply responding to the experience of that culture. The claims of the power of the witch doctor may not stand up to external scrutiny, nor might the eclipse of the sun really precede a major trauma, but this does not stop people believing what they have heard from the earlier generations who are the 'authority figures' in their society. In some instance the witch doctor may be seen to heal the sick or cast a spell; the eclipse may precede a major trauma. However, this may be said to be in just the same way that gifts were left for you by 'Father Christmas' when you were a child. In effect the beliefs are generated by the experiences, myths and legends of the culture.

So, when we try to focus on what people think and feel about a given situation we are faced with the challenge of trying to understand the influences that might have shaped a person's perception of the world. This applies whether you are endeavouring to understand a philosophical viewpoint or whether you are planning to undertake a research study to determine what people feel in a given situation.

Knowledge development: voice of authority

All the processes associated with thinking and feeling about the world around us are shaped, often unconsciously, by our experiences of the world around us and in that world there are wide-ranging influences and experiences that serve to shape our thoughts, not least the 'authority' figures we experience. The first figures of authority most of us knew were our parents: they shaped our early views of the world. In due course they were replaced by teachers and lecturers as we moved through the educational system and now, for many of us, the authority figures are our managers at work.

If you reflect on the voice of authority, consider for a moment how as a child and young person you were prepared to accept as 'fact' what the 'authority' told you about the world. Gradually, as your own life experiences expanded you might have felt more confident about challenging what you were told by these people 'in authority'. You only have to consider the classic teenage rebellion in the western world to recognise that! We live in a culture where the education system encourages people to be questioning and challenging. However, it is not always so easy or appropriate to question authority figures and it is for this reason that some authors have suggested that a further source of knowledge in health care is that of 'authority' – the people who have developed wisdom from professional experience providing a cumulative 'knowledge' that is passed down from generation to generation. One of the questions facing the research-aware health care practitioner today is to question the source of knowledge that provides the base for advice from authority figures – is it based on factual knowledge or is it based on their own experiences or philosophies of life?

Knowledge development: using observation

When considering our own experiences and the feelings that arise from them we need to recognise the potential limitations of the world in which an individual lives. As we look at the world around us we might conclude that what we see is indicative of the world at large. In health care it is very important that we use our senses to observe what is happening around us and it is those observations that cause us to act on behalf of our patients and clients. For example, if we saw someone obviously upset we would go and comfort them.

It is possible that some days you might go to work and see a lot of people who are upset; certainly if you work in health care you will see a lot of people with health problems. It would be very easy on the basis of this observation to conclude that 'everybody' is upset or ill but this would not be true – only the people you have seen on that day were upset or ill and in the world at large there are many people who are perfectly happy and healthy. This is an important point for, as you will see later, researchers are commonly concerned with the issue of bias in their studies. *Bias* is defined as any unintended influence on research that may distort the findings.

Linked with this we need to make a distinction between those dimensions of human nature that can be directly observed when compared with those we cannot 'see'. We cannot observe what people are thinking although we can observe patterns of behaviour that may allow us to infer what those thoughts may be. This is not so straightforward: for example, you might observe the smiling face of the man knocking at the front door of your house and assume that he is happy. However, this is not always the case: travelling salesmen for example, are advised that smiling will help to build a rapport with their customers and may therefore increase sales. The smile on the man's face may not be indicative of internal happiness if he knocks on your door having failed to sell any goods in the previous thirty houses. So, whilst observation might contribute towards our knowledge development we must be cautious again of the context in which we are making such observations.

Now we have introduced a note of caution, we must not underestimate the power of observation when gathering data in research; indeed, as we will see in subsequent chapters, the word 'observation' is widely used to indicate a range of ways in which data are collected in research. This is commonly used in the context of *empirical* research which refers to data collected by using the senses.

There are numerous instances where observations may serve to give a clear indication of the human state. For example, during the course of my observations I might observe blood tests in a laboratory and be able to see the micro-organisms that have been cultured from the blood; I might observe someone who has been running and note they were breathless; or I might observe a crowd of patients in a hospital waiting room and note patterns of behaviour as they talked to each other and moved along the queue to see the doctor, nurse or physiotherapist during the course of my observations.

The more complex the situations we observe, the harder it is to draw out the 'facts'. If we continue with our example from above it may be relatively straightforward exercise to observe one set of the micro-organism in one blood sample. However, if this observation was extended and I was asked to identify all the different types of blood cells, my ability to focus would be challenged. If I was to observe that someone who had been running was breathless again this would not be so complicated, but if I was to try to analyse that further and wanted to determine why that breathlessness had occurred I would need to introduce a range of other observations such as pulse rate, blood pressure and so on.

In both of the examples above I could focus on a single 'case' and a number of issues – repeated blood tests or repeated physiological measures of people who had been running – to build up a 'picture' of what is happening in each situation. In the last case, the observation of the crowd of people in the hospital waiting area is more challenging as I am focusing on a group rather than on an individual unit or person. This is clearly more complex than my single observations above. The complexities of observing the world around us need further consideration and this is the major consideration when looking at knowledge development from a 'scientific' perspective.

Knowledge development: the scientific perspective

Scientists will state that their work involves developing knowledge about 'facts' and that these facts represent 'truths' which can be contrasted with 'assumptions' which are not demonstrated to be true. In looking for the truth of a given situation a scientist will seek to challenge any assumptions and look for certainty, or an ability to predict the occurrence of particular events.

To illustrate this consider the oft-cited story of the chicken in the farmyard being fed on a daily basis by the farmer's wife. The 'assumption' for this chicken is that each day when the farmer's wife appears it will be fed. Then one day the farmer's wife appears and wrings the chicken's neck. The 'truth' for the farmer's wife is that she has been feeding the chicken to fatten it up for Sunday lunch; the chicken 'assumed' a level of care but did not look beyond this and so, one day, the assumptions proved incorrect.

A scientific perspective of knowledge development is based on a premiss that if we can predict what will happen in a given situation we are dealing in facts; if we cannot predict this we are dealing in assumptions. To predict what will happen in a given situation we need to be able to identify the *cause and effect* of the observation.

For example, let us consider a time at which people were finding out how the body works. At this time someone would have observed that people exposed to a frightening experience, perhaps a loud bang, react in the same way and seem to exhibit a set of physiological symptoms. To confirm this they could measure physiological reaction, for example heart rate, skin colour and pupil size. They might conclude that if exposed to a fright an individual's heart would beat faster, skin would become pale and the pupils in the eyes would dilate. As more and more people were observed to have this reaction following a fright, confidence develops in the 'facts' that were identified by observation.

Other people may question these observations and set out to challenge the conclusion. In this instance the challengers might proceed to expose a number of other people to a frightening situation and proceed to measure the physiological response. If they too found the same response to a frightening situation they might begin to accept the physiological response as 'factual' knowledge. These observations provide more evidence to support the claim that exposure to a frightening situation will cause a predictable physiological response.

However, these people are only reporting what they see; that is, they are *describing* the situation they observe. They cannot say with certainty that everybody exposed to a frightening situation will respond in exactly the same way. (If you doubt this statement, refer back to the story of the chicken above – just because it was fed every day when the farmer's wife appeared did not mean that it was going to be fed every day thereafter.)

It might be that some people who had not been observed might react differently to the experience of a fright. In such a situation these people will have to consider ways in which they can find out if what they are reporting is based on their own observations only or whether there are ways they can develop their observations to enable them to say with some certainty that this response is a 'fact'. To establish the basis of the facts they will need to look for ways to measure *cause and effect*. This will require the use of specific measures that will form the base not only of the original research but also enable anyone interested in challenging the findings to replicate the research.

Once such measures are available it may be suggested that anyone trained to use the measure can do so. If a proposed relationship between cause and effect is stated and measures to determine this identified, we might expect consistency in response if there is a relationship between cause and effect. Thus, again a simple example, we might propose that the rate at which a heart is beating can be measured by counting the pulse rate in the wrist. This may also be said to be a *valid* measure because it is measuring what it is supposed to measure, the pulse rate *is* indicative of the rate at which the heart is beating. If the measure was *reliable* we might expect that it would consistently produce the same result – if the pulse was counted over a one minute period this would be indicative of the heart rate in that time. Moreover this would be a consistent measure in that the rate would be the same regardless of whether an experienced cardiologist or an inexperienced student nurse was counting at the same time. The measure of pulse in this situation is said to be *reliable* because, when replicated, it yields the same outcome. We will return to the concepts of *reliability* and *validity* later in the text.

So, in contrast to our own unstructured observations of the world around us we are introducing some structure into our observations and using means of *measuring* what we see as a basis for our reports; moreover it has been suggested that such measures could be used repeatedly to measure the same phenomenon, in our example pulse rate. Research approaches drawing on structured observations in this way are said to be empirical – that is, they have relied on observations. We will return to these concepts in Chapter 8.

Knowledge development: abstract to concrete

So far it has been suggested that the development of knowledge may be linked to ways of reasoning, influenced by figures of authority in sharing their knowledge and the influence of our own experiences by using observations to, at one level, observe the world around us and at another to differentiate the facts of a situation from the assumptions. It is these different ways of exploring situations that gives a structure to approaches to research in health care.

This interpretation gives a framework of knowledge development that can be seen in Figure 5.1. In this figure the potential range of knowledge development has been illustrated on a continuum from abstract to concrete to try to illustrate the distinction between knowledge developed on the basis of reasoning which offers an interpretation of the world around us when compared with knowledge developed through observation and measurement which is more concrete. Some authors refer to information or data collected and developed at the abstract end of the continuum as 'soft' whilst knowledge developed at the concrete end is said to be 'hard'. We will return to this notion of soft and hard data later.

Our own experiences of life will determine the extent to which we move in a world dominated by abstract knowledge development or by concrete knowledge development. Consider, for example, the distinction between the experiences of the world of the creative writer and the scientist. The world of the writer is dominated by presenting interpretations of the world through story-telling, whilst the world of the scientist is dominated by looking for facts under the microscope. Both contribute much to the

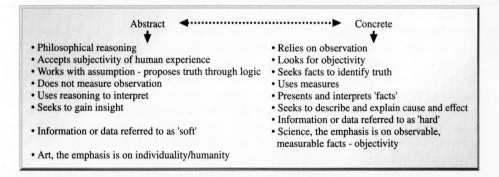

Figure 5.1 Knowledge development: abstract to concrete.

world in which we live, yet the approach in so doing is quite different. In this world the writer will appreciate the results of the work of the science in the development of new products, and the scientist will appreciate the interpretation of the writer when looking for relaxation from the normal routine of work. Consequently, some might suggest that the abstract end of the continuum represents the artistic end of human endeavour in which the emphasis is on the subjectivity of human experience, whilst the concrete end represents the scientific implications of human endeavour in which knowledge is developed through observation and measurement and is thus objective.

One of the challenges facing health care workers today is to draw out the sources of knowledge guiding their practice at a given time. Our approach to care may be influenced by both poles of the continuum in Figure 5.1 in that we are concerned with both the art and science of caring, that is the endeavour to gain insight into the human state and the need to understand many facts concerning cause and effect of problems we deal with every day.

Awareness of such differing perspectives is important when you are approaching research studies as the ways in which people view the world will influence the way in which they view approaches to research. These principles underpin two differing approaches to research that we referred to above as qualitative and quantitative approaches to research.

Qualitative and quantitative approaches to research

The discussion on knowledge development has relevance for research when we begin to consider the different approaches that may be adopted by researchers to develop knowledge through the process of research. In the section above a distinction was made between the creativity of art, the logic of philosophy and the factual knowledge that may be derived from structured observation as distinct from our own general observations of the world around us. In research the emphasis is on the development of factual knowledge but, in developing this knowledge base a number of influences may shape the approach that is adopted in the research and, to some extent, fuels the debate about what constitutes fact.

To illustrate this let us consider a situation in which a nurse wants to understand how his or her patients feel about the treatment they are receiving for their health care problem. He or she could do this in an open way in which he or she simply asks them to tell in their own words what they feel about their experiences. The information, or *data*, collected will be in the form of words, the responses that people gave to the question about being a patient in a hospital ward. These people have told the nurse what *they feel* about the situation.

Another way the nurse could have collected the data would have been to devise a short questionnaire that asked the patients to respond in very specific ways to the questions asked. For example he or she might have asked questions such as 'Were you comfortable in hospital?', 'Did you get enough information from the staff?' and so on. These questions could demand a simple 'yes' or 'no' answer. In this situation the data collected could be counted. For example if fifty patients answered the questionnaires the nurse could count the number of people who said yes to specific questions and the number who said no. Thus the data are said to be numerical. In this case the nurse has identified areas that *he or she feels* the patients would identify as areas of concern.

Whilst the example above is a simple illustration it serves to indicate the distinction in many textbooks between what is described as qualitative research and what is described as quantitative research. *Qualitative* approaches to research are, broadly speaking, those approaches in which the information, or data, is generated in words by the *respondents*, that is the people participating as research *subjects*. The data may come directly from the subjects themselves or generated by the researcher observing the subject in a given situation. So in this approach, when the time comes to analyse the data the researcher will be analysing the 'words' generated.

In the second case referred to above we suggested the interviewer may collect the information in a more structured way using a pre-set questionnaire. In this case the researcher has set the framework and the respondents will indicate the extent to which they agree with set questions by giving a 'yes' or 'no' response to the question asked. The researcher will count the number of responses to each question. In this case the range of data that will be collected is fixed by the researcher who has set the questions. The responses can be categorised in numerical form.

Newcomers to research may be confused by the various claims about the benefits or otherwise of each type of approach to research but the important point to remember is that the type of research adopted by a researcher will depend on the questions to be asked. To illustrate this a little more let us consider how factual knowledge is developed.

Developing factual knowledge

As this book is designed for nurses and health care workers it is safe to assume that most readers will have a good working knowledge of how the body works – the anatomy and physiology of body systems. If you cast your mind back a few years you might remember that there was a time when you were not so knowledgeable. You might have struggled to understand how the cell works and, perhaps, at times, questioned the need for such detailed knowledge if your career was to be dealing with whole people not just parts of people! However, as your knowledge improved you would have begun to make connections between how the cells work and how in joining together they make organs and ultimately body systems.

You might have looked at models of body organs and traced the connections between the organs in blood vessels and nerve tissue to understand that the body is in fact an integrated whole. If you had access to sophisticated models or perhaps computer packages you would have been able to test your evolving knowledge about the body, trying to see what happened in different circumstances, in other words, by testing your knowledge as it developed. Computer models allow you, for example, to see what happens in imaginary situations when you try out an idea. Alternatively you might have undertaken some exercises with your colleagues and, for example,

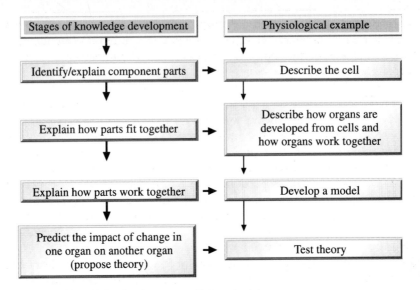

Figure 5.2 Stages of knowledge development applied to physiology.

measured heart rate and respiratory rate before and after sending your colleagues to run a hundred metres or so. In this case you were testing your ideas or knowledge base of the circulatory and respiratory systems in action. You might have formulated a 'theory' that running will increase the heart and respiratory rates.

If we were to draw this process of learning out in diagrammatic form we might suggest that the process you went through in developing your knowledge of physiology followed the steps in Figure 5.2. We can relate the stages outlined in the figure to research. The purpose of research is to develop knowledge, using some of the same principles we used unconsciously when we developed our knowledge about physiology, so let us think about how knowledge is developed through research.

When we undertake research we are aiming to develop new knowledge. Unlike our physiology example, it is not always easy to predict what might happen in a given situation. For example, whilst we might accept as 'fact' the way we have described above of how the circulatory and respiratory systems will respond to exercise, there are still aspects of body function that remain unknown. Scientists continue to explore the components of cells, try to explain how they fit together and develop models that will enable them to predict 'what might happen if', but the level of knowledge is such that sometimes the predictions proposed in their theories do not always work. A good example of this is the way in which scientists try to understand how viruses and other diseases affect the body. As knowledge develops in relation to one aspect of the disease process caused by a certain virus, so another comes along to challenge this initiative. In response to the question 'why?' in some aspects of research the researcher might get an answer to one question, but yet another question raises its head. Consequently much of the knowledge development today is evolutionary rather than revolutionary. However, this should not reduce the awareness of researchers to the possibilities open to them, for an important point is that research is a *dynamic process* in which the answer to one question leads to a need to rethink the basis of knowledge developed earlier. This is a very important concept and the reason why the issue of context in the development of knowledge was discussed earlier in this chapter.

It is important to recognise that just because something has been identified at a point of history it does not always mean that it is the 'truth'. New knowledge from other sources or a new possibility when examining information opens up challenges to accepted patterns of knowledge. This applies equally to knowledge developed in the western world in the twentieth century as it does to the difference between the West and other cultures in terms of the way we observe the world around us. It is just as easy for knowledge generated by earlier research to become fixed as the truth as it is for personal views of authoritarian knowledge to become embedded into our minds as 'truth' – in other words research can lead to ritualistic or traditional patterns as well as other sources of knowledge!

Consider, for example, the case of duodenal ulcers. Many health professionals who have been working in health care for some years will be able to tell how it was thought that stomach ulceration was caused by factors such as stress and smoking, and that the prescribed treatment to alleviate this problem was to treat with rest and antacids to relieve the gastric irritation caused by high acid levels. Now it is widely accepted that the majority of stomach ulcers are caused by a bacterium, *Helicobacter pylori*, and can be treated with an antibiotic – quite a radical change in perception. This 'new insight' came from researchers constantly challenging the accepted way of looking at things: new knowledge was derived by placing such a challenge. It was not accepted widely 'overnight' – as with all new knowledge, the sceptics continued to rely on old knowledge to inform their practices. This is not unusual with any new treatments in health care since practitioners want to be convinced about the source of knowledge and to distinguish facts from assumptions.

So let us return to the ways in which knowledge is developed and consider these from the perspective of developing knowledge through research. It has been noted above (see Figure 5.1) that knowledge may be perceived from differing perspectives. Whilst it is acknowledged that one perspective seeks to understand and interpret the world around us, accounting for the subjectivity of human experience, another focuses on the development of factual knowledge that can be measured in a quantifiable way. The approaches adopted can be identified in the stages of knowledge development outlined in Figure 5.3.

Broadly speaking the stages of knowledge development can be associated with the differing orientation of qualitative and quantitative research. Stage 1 involves the identification of concepts or ideas relating to a specific area of interest. So, for example, if you wanted to find out how people feel if a relative has been seriously injured you might simply ask them that question. As a result of your enquiry you might identify that the people you talk to have similar feelings which you label as 'why me?' or 'disbelief' and so on. These words may have been derived from your discussion in that the relatives you interviewed commonly used them in the conversation to describe how they felt.

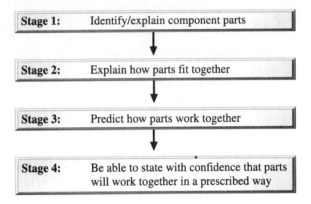

Figure 5.3 Stages of knowledge development.

If you then wanted to move to stage 2 of knowledge development you might try to explain how these concepts 'fit' together. You might note, for example, an observation that people who demonstrate disbelief have greater difficulty in adapting to the injuries to their relative. However, you would only be describing what you had *interpreted* from the data – you would not be able to state this was the case in every similar situation. If you wanted to demonstrate that you would need to move to stage 3 of knowledge development and predict that, in the situation observed, certain things might happen. In other words you would be *proposing* a relationship between the concepts which is leading to formulation of a theory of relatives' response to serious injury. If you were able to test your propositions you might then be able to say with confidence that, in a situation where an accident occurred to relatives, then certain reactions may be expected – in other words you could *prescribe* the response to that situation.

When dealing with this model of knowledge development from the point of view of feeling and emotions, this idea can be quite difficult and it may be easier to expand this explanation by using a physiological example. Take, for example, many of the drugs that we work with today in health care and consider the origins of knowledge about these drugs. At some point in time it was observed that certain substances identified from plants had certain effects on the body and so were useful when people demonstrated certain physical symptoms. Such observations would have been taken in ignorance of how drugs work and even what was wrong with the people suffering problems, and so may be located at stage 1 of the knowledge development model.

Over time there would have been a wide acceptance that these drugs had a specific reaction and people would have wanted to try to explain why they worked as they did. To do this they would look at component parts of the drug and the body systems to determine how they interacted, this is stage 2 of the model above (Figure 5.3). Once such component parts had been identified it would be possible to make a prediction that in certain situations this drug would produce a specific reaction (stage 3 of knowledge development). To be sure of this the research team would need to

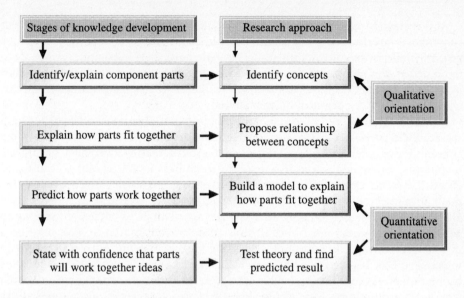

Figure 5.4 Stages of knowledge development, research approaches and orientation.

propose a relationship between cause and effect, to ensure the ways they were observing that cause and effect were free from bias, and finally the research team might be able to say with confidence that if a person has a certain problem the drug would have this effect. This is illustrated in Figure 5.4.

Why the conflict with qualitative/quantitative approaches to research ?

Many research texts and journal articles seek to justify a particular orientation to research as being the 'right' way to address the question. However, as was noted in Chapter 3, the question you ask will largely determine the approach you need to develop. For example, if you are a pharmacist undertaking a research project into a new drug you will of course being interested how people who take the drug feel about it, but this will not tell you whether the drug is safe to administer or prescribe on a day-to-day basis. Consequently if you were exploring the latter issue you would undertake a quantitatively orientated study that will indicate whether it is safe to prescribe the drug. Researchers using a quantitative ordination are more orientated towards being able to identify the impact of certain concepts as a generalisable phenomenon. That is they want to know the extent to which the findings from a study sample can be *generalised* to the population from which the sample was taken. This has an impact on the way the research design is developed as you will see in the chapters that follow. In research that has a qualitative orientation, researchers argue that in identifying concepts or feelings, for example, they do not need to approach large numbers of people.

At this stage it may be useful to note that, although individual researchers might subscribe firmly to either a qualitative or a quantitative research approach this generally reflects their area of interest. The epidemiologist, for example, will be more interested in demographic trends as that is the focus of his or her work. The counsellor in health care might be more interested in the intensity of feeling generated in specific client groups which consist of only small numbers.

In health care research both qualitative and quantitative approaches to research serve a useful purpose. Qualitative research deals in feelings, emotions and unearthing concepts for research which help inform practice by increasing awareness. In contrast quantitative orientated research is designed to address issues relating to cause and effect. Some may claim that quantitative research represents science while the qualitative research is too subjective to be taken seriously as an approach to research. However, overall it may be suggested that the approaches are 'different', seeking to address different questions. In health care we do of course need to have hard facts of which treatment will work most effectively for our patients, but we also need to understand how people feel and the concerns that may impact on the care. In some health care professions the level of knowledge development is such that most research work is located in stages 3 and 4 of the knowledge development model outlined above in Figure 5.3; however, in other professions so little is known about the impact of care that knowledge development is still firmly located in stages 1 and 2 – those of concept identification.

In the next chapter the difference between quantitative and qualitative research when planning a research study will be considered in more detail.

Triangulation

A number of studies in health care research incorporate the principles of both qualitative and quantitative research. This enables researchers to consider the phenomenon under study for different perspectives and so contributes towards developing a more 'complete' picture. For example, the pharmacist referred to above may be interested in the overall impact of the drug in terms of physiological outcome using a quantitative orientation to measure the impact of the drug on the overall treatment of the patient. However, increasingly people undertaking such studies are interested in looking at the effect of the drug in qualitative terms – does it, for example, help improve the patient's quality of life? To explore this could require a more qualitatively orientated approach. Consequently a researcher may mix the approaches to research. A term used to describe mixed approaches to data collection and data analysis is triangulation. *Triangulation* is described as the use of more than one method of collecting or interpreting data.

ACTIVITY _____

- Consider your own area of work and, alongside each source of knowledge listed below, note an aspect of your own learning that has been influenced by it:

philosophical reasoning   ....

....

influence of authority   ....

....

your own observation   ....

....

scientific knowledge   ....

....

- Refer back to the area you noted you might like to research (Activity in Chapter 3). Note whether you think this has a qualitative orientation or a quantitative orientation.

Summary

In this chapter the issues relating to differing approaches to developing knowledge and the implications of these in research terms have been discussed. The issues discussed in this chapter are important in helping you to decide what you are trying to achieve when you are planning to develop a research study. The further reading at the end of the chapter offers a range of literature that will help you to examine this subject further.

Further reading

Berger, R.M. and Patchup, M.A. (1988) *Planning for Research. A Guide for the Helping Professions*, Sage, London.

Brockopp, D.Y. and Hastings-Tolsma, M.T. (1995) *Fundamentals of Nursing Research*, 2nd edn, Jones & Bartlett, Boston.

Carr, L.T. (1994) 'The strengths and weaknesses of quantitative and qualitative research: what method for nursing?', *Journal of Advanced Nursing*, vol. 20, no. 4, pp. 716–721.

Chapman, J. (1991) 'Research – What it is and what it is not', in Perry, A. and Jolley M., *Nursing – A Knowledge Base for Practice*, Edward Arnold, London, Ch. 2.

Clarke, E. (1991) *Research Awareness Module 2 Sources of Nursing Knowledge*, Distance Learning Centre, South Bank Polytechnic (South Bank University), London.

Cormack, D.F.S. (1991) *The Research Process in Nursing*, 2nd edn, Blackwell Scientific, Oxford.

Corner, J. (1991) 'In search of more complete answers to research questions. Quantitative vs qualitative research methods: is there a way forward?', *Journal of Advanced Nursing*, vol. 16, pp. 718–727.

Cowman, S. (1993) 'Triangulation: a means of reconciling in nursing research', *Journal of Advanced Nursing*, vol. 18, pp. 788–792.

Duffy, M.E. (1985) 'Designing nursing research: the qualitative – quantitative debate', *Journal of Advanced Nursing*, vol. 10, pp. 225–232.

Fawcett, J. and Downs, F. (1992) *The Relationship of Theory and Research*, F.A. Davies & Company, Philadelphia.

Gaarder, J. (1995) *Sophie's World. A Novel About the History of Philosophy*, Phoenix House, London.
Robinson, K. and Vaughan, B. (1992) *Knowledge for Nursing Practice*, Butterworth-Heinemann, Oxford.

6   The research process outlined

This chapter will give an overview of the various stages that a researcher will go through when planning a research study. This, sometimes known as the 'research process', involves several stages of careful planning and implementation of plans. The chapter is designed to give a source of quick reference rather than to be a definitive guide as to how to do research. However, it is anticipated that by the end of the chapter you should be able to give a *broad outline of the research process.*

Subsequent chapters will give more detail relating to the research design issues referred to here and cross-reference will be made to these as appropriate. Readers with specific research projects in mind are also recommended to the further reading noted at the end of this and subsequent chapters.

The process covers the same general areas regardless of whether the overall research design is qualitative or quantitative in orientation. The main stages are outlined in general terms as specified in Table 6.1, which also outlines how each stage may vary depending on whether the research design is to be qualitative or quantitative.

Defining the research problem

At the beginning of a research study there is a need to clarify the area of study and make a clear statement of what is seen to be the research problem. Very often when reading research reports it may appear that the researchers have simply decided what they will study and begun their work in that area without any great difficulty. In reality, as noted in earlier chapters, most researchers start with a general idea of the problem area. This is subsequently refined to give a specific focus to the study. This refinement is achieved by a critical analysis of the subject area, based on both personal knowledge of the subject and the information obtained from the literature available. Quite frequently, researchers will also have discussed their ideas in some depth with supervisors or colleagues to help clarify their research ideas at the outset.

Following this period of consideration, discussion and review the researcher should be in a position to clarify the area for research, that is to define the problem area. This preparation time is seen to be a very important phase in the research process and can be quite a lengthy process.

Table 6.1 Stages of the research process in qualitative and quantitative research

Stages of research	Qualitative research	Quantitative research
Defining the problem	Statement of problem area	Statement of problem area
Searching the literature	May precede study and be ongoing; or may follow initial data collection	Precedes data collection and ongoing
The research design	States research questions or aims	States aims or hypothesis
	Descriptive, exploratory	Descriptive, exploratory correlation, experimental designs
Techniques of data collection	Interview, observation, questionnaire, diaries, records	Questionnaire, interview Observation, records
	Structure to question generates data in words	Structure to question generates predetermined categories of data that can be numerically calculated
Population and samples	May use small samples – does not rely on random sampling procedures	Sampling tends to be large, using random sampling procedures if possible
Pilot study	To develop approaches of data collection	To develop research instruments and test approach to data collection
Data analysis	Content analysis of words to identify concepts and themes	Descriptive statistics to indicate trends Inferential statistics to infer implications
Ethical permission	Required if patient/client contact in NHS	Required if patient/client contact in NHS
Access	Permission to access respondents required	Permission to access respondents required
The research report	Identifies methodology, discusses themes	Identifies methodology, discusses findings in context of statistical analysis and implications for larger population
	Strengths and limitations of research approach noted	Strengths and limitations of research approach noted
Dissemination	Important to increase insight and contribute towards knowledge development	Important to identify trends or facts as appropriate

Once the problem area is clearly identified the researcher may move on to the next stage, searching the literature. It should be noted here that some qualitative research approaches do not review the literature at the outset; the reasons for this will be discussed further in Chapter 7.

Searching the literature

This stage can be broken down into two components, the literature search and the literature review. The former involves the mechanism involved in finding the data in the first instance, the latter involves reading and drawing conclusions from the literature.

Why undertake a literature review?

The purpose of undertaking a literature review is to identify the need to undertake the research in the first instance and secondly to inform the researcher about potential research designs that could be adopted. If there was an evident gap in the literature this might indicate a need to start at the base of the knowledge development pyramid and begin the process by identifying the concepts concerned from a qualitative perspective. Alternatively, if someone had already completed a sound study on the topic previously there may be a need to replicate it from the perspective of your own work in health care.

The more knowledge that can be gathered in searching the literature the easier it is for the researcher to identify which specific areas would benefit from further study. If the researcher has, for example, started thinking about research in a broad subject area such as communication in health care he or she will find, in only a preliminary skim of available literature, that there is a need to reduce the area of interest to provide a specific focus for the research study. For example, he or she may decide to study a more clearly defined area such as communication in the health care team. If this option was chosen, the volume of available literature on the subject would be markedly reduced and consequently the practitioner may be better able to clarify ideas for a research study.

Searching the literature can also help indicate which research design would be most appropriate for the study. Information on the research methods utilised in studies undertaken into the subject area will help in this, for generally the strengths and weaknesses of research methodology are discussed in research reports.

Reading literature also helps avoid duplication or 'rediscovering the wheel'. Unless the researchers are aware of studies previously undertaken, they will not know whether their study is an original piece of work. It may be a wasted effort to plan and implement a research study, only to find at a later date that all the work has been done before and the evidence of that work is more than sufficient for practice developments.

The possibility of *replicating research studies* is another aspect that can be considered when reading literature. Although one reason for searching literature is to avoid duplication there is much to be said in favour of replicating reported research projects, particularly if they are small-scale projects. In quantitative research approaches, for example, factors such as sample size contribute towards the ability of the researcher to be able to generalise the findings to a wide range of settings. The implications of sample sizes are discussed in more detail later in this chapter but it is worth emphasising that if a research study is undertaken with only a small sample it may not be appropriate to apply the findings in a variety of settings. This lack of ability to generalise findings can be a major problem for nurses and other health care workers looking for research on which to base their practices. However, as research is still a relatively new phenomenon for some health care practitioners many reported projects are still classed as small scale. The value of replication lies in the fact that if many small-scale research studies, exploring similar themes, were to result in similar findings then health care workers can be more confident about utilising such findings in different settings.

The literature search

The advent of computer technology has created a curious paradox for researchers searching for research literature in their area of study. On the one hand it has made life a lot easier in terms of the time spent in libraries. Only a very short time ago searching the literature meant spending a long time reviewing published indexes that were available on the library shelves. A common frustration with these indexes was that they were inevitably out of date by the time they reached the library shelves with even the most recent publication drawing on literature that was commonly several months old. Now, however, most health care libraries have ready access to computing facilities which use compact discs, the so-called CD-ROM (compact disc, read-only memory) system. The speed at which these can be updated and circulated to libraries means that health care staff who wish to search the literature can now readily access records of the most up-to-date publications in their field of interest. Moreover, even with a simple home computer it is possible through networking systems to access a wide range of bibliographic indexes.

Despite these advantages there are some problems with the availability of literature. The first problem relates to the accessibility of journal articles that are cited. If these are not readily available in your library you may have difficulty tracking them down. The second is that it is not uncommon for a large number of references to be written in a language other than your own – quite frustrating if it looks like the exact piece of work you require for your project. Another problem is that all registered work is cited on such databases – for example a range of references may refer to M.Phil. or Ph.D. theses in different countries. These are not readily or easily available, although some publishers are endeavouring to increase the availability of such material over computerised networks. Overall, however, it can be very frustrating if reading the abstracts on the CD-ROM printout you find that the perfect piece of work of relevance to your study is a North American Ph.D. that is only available from the archives of that university.

Given the increase in the range of professional publications you might find that searching the literature results in your being inundated with references appropriate to your topic. So, as you begin your literature search it is advisable, especially at undergraduate level, to set some parameters on the range of literature you might draw on. However, you are not advised to do this alone – it is certainly something you should discuss with your supervisor as the parameter set will be very specific to your own study.

The opposite problem is the one where there is very little literature on the topic. In this instance there may be no stronger incentive to undertake the research as such a situation may indicate a gap in knowledge.

The skills required to use the CD-ROM systems are beyond the scope of this book and are better taught by librarians who can give you hands-on experience of the computer. Consequently rather than exploring the issue here, if you are not familiar with how to use computers to search literature you will need to go to your own academic library and find this out.

Reading literature

Reading the literature is the point at which you actually get down to focusing your research and read or review the material you have. The first question to ask is 'how much do I read?'. As you will see in Chapter 11 where the literature review is discussed in more depth, there is no clear answer to this and it is perhaps an issue that, if in doubt, you should discuss with your supervisor.

When reviewing the literature your reading here needs to be 'active', not just simply a skim read and discard. We will return to this in more detail in Chapter 11 where the art of writing a literature review is considered and compared with a critique of the literature – a more critical review of research material. However, at this stage you should note that it is important that you do not simply file away your thoughts in an inaccessible manner. One way of avoiding this, and again one that is relatively easily developed either manually or on a computer, is to keep an overall record of research related to your topic.

It is important that all health care practitioners are able to read research reports in a critical manner. Obviously the more critical the reader, the better able he or she is to judge the quality of the research studies undertaken. This is a very important point for it must be acknowledged that not all research reported is good research and the newcomer to the subject needs to be alert to this fact. Just because a research project has been reported in the professional press, this does not mean that the findings should be adopted in every clinical area. Many factors contribute towards the quality of a good research project and professional journals have differing criteria as to what is seen as acceptable material for publication. You should clarify the status of the sources of information when reading and take care not to assume that all published research is good research.

To be able to read a research report effectively the nurse or other health care worker needs some insight into the research process. Consequently it is felt that this chapter provides a source of reference for anyone wishing to learn the broad areas of research considered when examining research reports.

Keeping records of literature reviewed

Whatever the reason for undertaking a literature search it is essential to keep note of the source of reference material. This is a practical tip that is often overlooked when searching for information. Keeping accurate records which summarises reading is a very good habit to get into from the outset of your research. No doubt there are some people who have the capacity of instant recall but unfortunately they are few and far between. For the majority it is advisable not to place too much reliance on memory when approaching a detailed literature search. It certainly helps avoid the frustration of being unable to relocate a piece of vital information that could be in any one of many books or journals.

There are an increasing number of computer packages available that enable you to keep your own records of references if you have ready access to a computer. You can do this in 'tables' format on most personal computers or you can get bibliographic packages which will enable you to transfer all the data you received from a CD-ROM search to your own file. If you can do this it will save you a lot of time and effort but if you do not have ready access to a computer system you can choose a number of ways to keep records, such as an alphabetical index book or a card file. The important thing is that whatever way you choose you should keep your records complete and up to date – most researchers will tell you of their frustration when they have failed to keep records accurately of having to start from scratch again to find their information.

The information you keep should include the complete, correct reference of the book or journal, which involves using the headings listed in Figure 6.1. In addition, the reference key words or descriptors can be noted to cross-reference your record with other material. This is useful when you want to cross-reference another theme or topic. For example you might be undertaking a study on pain in chronic illness. In the course of your reading you identify different issues relating to age and ethnicity. Thus if you were reading an article that had implications for pain in childhood your descriptor might be 'pain in childhood'. There might also be issues relating to pain in ethnic groups in the same article so your descriptor would be ethnicity. This way allows you to develop groups of literature that have specific theme references over and above your broad subject area. Such cross-referencing may not seem necessary if you are working with a small amount of literature but you might find that once you get beyond reading say twenty articles relating to your topic, your memory relating to the content of each may not be perfect.

In addition, if you use several libraries, it is worth noting on the card whether you have your own copy of the reference or if not, exactly where the journal or book was located, so that you can relocate it as and when you want it.

Time required to do a literature review

Another point is not to underestimate the time required to spend on searching and reading literature before beginning the actual research study. Whilst I indicated above

Journal reference

```
Author:
Date of publication:
Title of article:
Journal title:
Volume no.; issue no.; page nos:
Location of journal/article:
Key words/descriptors:
```

Book reference

```
Author/Editor (Ed.):
Year of publication:
Title (edition):
Place of publication:
Publisher:
Location (which library, class mark):
Key words/Descriptors ISBN:
```

Figure 6.1 Information to be included in a card index.

that searching the literature is much more straightforward with the advent of the CD-ROM facility, the time taken to get hold of articles may not be any quicker if it relies on sending to other libraries for copies of articles or texts.

Designing the study

It has been suggested above that, depending on the overall purpose of the study and the questions the researcher wants to answer, a research study may fall into the category of qualitative or quantitative design. For example, if you wanted to find out how people feel about their chronic illness you would be advised to consider research that has a qualitative orientation. In contrast if you wanted to find out whether dark winter days caused depression you might want to undertake a more quantitative orientation in which you might seek to measure cause and effect, measuring daylight hours against the mood of the individual.

Following the review of the literature, the researcher may find that some of the original ideas for the research project have been clarified or redirected. The problem area outlined at the beginning of the study may be modified or redefined and aims for the research project are identified. However, before you can begin to collect data you need to consider fully what approach you are going to take in your research.

The factors that might help you in your decision making here will include the following:

1. Whether the overall 'problem' or research question leads to a qualitative or quantitative study.

2. The range of research already completed on the topic and whether the published research answers all the questions in relation to your area of interest.
3. Any gaps in the literature in terms of areas of study completed.
4. Any methodological gaps – perhaps the area of interest has been examined from one perspective only.
5. Time and resources available to complete the study.

Considering these questions will help focus your study. Any evident gaps in the literature in terms of knowledge base can be readily identified and lend support to the need to undertake your research. However, methodological gaps can also be identified. For example, when reading the literature you might find your area of interest has been well examined from a quantitative perspective yet the qualitative dimension has perhaps not been so well considered.

Other considerations in deciding the research approach discussed in Chapter 4 include the implications of time and resources available. It was noted that the size of the project will clearly be influenced by these limitations and, from this perspective, original ideas for research may need to be trimmed down to make a study more feasible. So, although you may want to undertake a large-scale study of your own client group both within your own area of work and in other NHS trusts as part of an undergraduate project, this may not be a realistic proposition in terms of time and resources available to you. In reality you may need to do a smaller project that is more realistic.

In terms of research design the broad umbrella terms of qualitative and quantitative research incorporate a number of research designs summarised in Figure 6.2. At one end of this continuum is descriptive research. As the aim of this approach is to describe, you should note that *qualitative research will always be descriptive* although other aspects of descriptive research may be quantitative. Other approaches to research will always be quantitative because the nature of measurement draws on numerical techniques. This includes comparative, correlational and experimental approaches. Researchers using a comparative approach will compare results for data collected from different groups of subjects or respondents to determine if there are differences between them.

As you will see in Chapter 8 the starting point for both correlational and experimental research is to formulate a *hypothesis*. A hypothesis is a statement of relationships between *variables* being studied. In research a variable is the term used to describe the characteristics or features of the objects or people in a research study. For example age, sex, level of education may be seen as variables that influence the way in which people may respond in a research study. The difference between the approaches can be seen in the way the study is developed. For example if a speech therapist wanted to ask other members of the health care team what they thought about the speech therapy service at a descriptive level, he or she might use a questionnaire survey to address that question. If this were to be developed as a correlational study he or she might formulate a hypothesis that states 'clinical staff referring to the speech therapy service on a weekly basis will hold a more positive view of the service than those staff using it less frequently'. To test this hypothesis

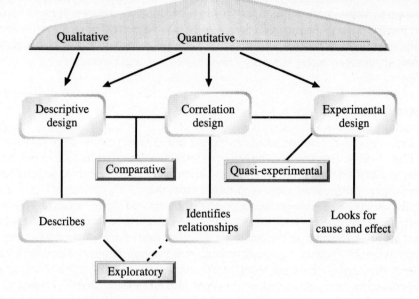

Figure 6.2 Broad categories of research design.

the therapist could send out a questionnaire to members of the health care team and, in addition to overall trends in the data collected, could look for relationships in the data collected. The experimental researcher, however, will take a more active role in developing the research by actually manipulating the situation in some way. So, for example, a speech therapist using an experimental approach may compare two different approaches to therapy and compare the effect of the two approaches. A quasi-experimental approach is used when the criteria for experimental design cannot be met (see Chapter 8).

Another term introduced in Figure 6.2 is *exploratory* research. This describes an approach in which researchers are beginning to explore a specific phenomenon and so is commonly used with descriptive research approaches, although sometimes it is used when developing correlational designs for exploratory purposes. As this is not a distinct approach in its own right we will not be referring to it as an independent entity.

There are some other research designs that have great relevance for health care which may draw on the principles of both qualitative and quantitative research. These include evaluation research, case studies and action research.

Evaluation research

Evaluation research is a research method which attempts to establish the value of a programme. It has become increasingly popular in recent years as practitioners question the value of their practices. Evaluation involves assessing progress against some predetermined measures and so can be used to determine the outcomes of health care programmes. The value is determined by whether or not the programme achieves its goals or meets the needs of users of the programme.

Case study

The term 'case study' will be familiar to most health care practitioners in that it has long been common practice for students to undertake an in-depth study of one patient as part of their learning process. These in-depth studies of care can be seen as having similar aspects to those of a research-based case study. This approach to research is quite frequently referred to as being on the opposite end of the spectrum from that of the survey approach. Surveys rely on an approach in which a large number of 'cases' are studied and a consensus view is drawn from the results of this study.

The case study focuses on one situation, or a limited number of people within a common situation such as the work-place, who are studied in depth in an attempt to give some meaning and additional insight into the subject under review.

In undertaking this in-depth analysis of a single situation the researcher can utilise a variety of techniques to gather information to obtain a more holistic picture. Information is gathered over a period of time, and therefore the research is put into the context of factors in the past and present rather than focusing on the here and now, which is a feature of survey research. Case studies can be useful in health care research for they are well suited to explore many situations that provide a focus in caring. For example, an in-depth study of one patient undergoing a new treatment regime will give insight into the individual's need and reactions. In providing this information the researcher may be able to give indicators for the future care of similar cases.

This approach to research also allows freedom in terms of the techniques that can be used to study the case. The researcher may use observational techniques but in addition may also use interviews or questionnaires when exploring the network of contacts related to the single case. For example, the researcher studying a student nurse as he or she progresses through his or her educational programme may wish to add the views of family, friends and colleagues to the study to give a more holistic picture.

The findings from a case study can lead to action if, for example, factors that affect an individual are identified and the response in a similar situation anticipated. This benefit can be important in health care. Finally, the wealth of information gained in a case study can generate ideas for future studies. Case studies can generate new concepts and theories for testing, unlike other forms of research when theories are tested.

The major disadvantage of case studies is the lack of ability to generalise findings to a variety of settings. In addition data gathered from one case study may be in conflict with data from another because of individual variations. This might happen if the researcher undertaking a case study of student nurses decided to examine more than one case, for example. Further disadvantages are related to the complexities of the research design. The researcher may have to decide whether to study a lot of aspects of the individual case superficially or a few aspects in depth. The wealth of knowledge that can be gathered in relation to any one case is enormous and can increase as the study progresses. Consequently there is a need to determine the boundaries of the study.

A final disadvantage of this method is that the costs of this type of research can be large compared with other approaches.

Action research

The focus of action research is on specific issues or problems identified in a local situation. An action plan is developed to introduce change to resolve the problems identified and subsequently the results are evaluated. Those people within the locality are involved in the research and because of this participation action research is seen as collaborative. Since the work is evaluated as it progresses, action research can be described as cyclical in nature. The problem-solving processes of assessment, planning, implementation and evaluation can be applied to this type of research.

In the assessment stage the specific problem would be identified. The researcher would plan a strategy to help solve the problem. In implementing the action plan he or she would begin to monitor the effects of the plan. Finally the whole process would be evaluated and the views of all participants incorporated into the evaluation. This evaluation would then form the basis of re-assessment as the whole process, or cycle, begins again with any modifications necessary being made.

In utilising this approach the researcher needs to consider wide-ranging issues. As with all research studies the overall aim of the research will help determine if this method is appropriate. The same point applies to the techniques utilised to collect data when evaluating the effects of the action.

The advantage of using this approach to research is that it offers a means of solving local problems. The emphasis on introducing and monitoring the effects of a change in the environment can help promote an interest in research amongst people who perhaps have not been involved in research studies before. Group participation in the research also helps to motivate and maintain interest. Also the research may be seen to be meaningful to participants as the results of changes made can be monitored closely at the point of action. This is unlike other research methods in which there is commonly a time lapse between completion of a research study and implementation of a preferred action plan based on the findings. The main disadvantage of using this method in research is that the findings cannot be generalised beyond the situation being examined.

Techniques of data collection

The techniques deployed in collecting data are described by researchers in their reports. Any problems encountered are usually noted and the newcomer to research is advised to read these carefully as recognition of the problems encountered by other researchers can help them avoid similar problems in their work. The techniques and design of research tools for collecting data are discussed in more detail in Chapter 9. The overall research design and aims of the research study will contribute towards the decisions made about which techniques to deploy in data collection.

Broadly speaking however, techniques of data collection can be categorised as those using the following:

1. Questionnaires.
2. Interviews.
3. Observation.
4. Records.

These approaches can be used in both qualitative and quantitative research although as you will see in Chapter 9, the way in which they are used will vary.

Population and samples

Any practitioner beginning a research study will need to consider the *population* and *sample* group that will be studied. A population is a group of subjects having common characteristics. For example all registered nurses may be seen as a population in a research study into nursing. A sample is seen as part of a whole. In research studies the population is the 'whole' that is to be studied whilst the sample selected for the study is seen as part of that whole. A *sample* is the group drawn from the population that actually participates in the study. The people participating in the sample group are sometimes referred to as *subjects, participants* or *respondents*.

As with other aspects of the research design, the way in which the sample is selected depends to a large extent on the overall research design. We will discuss this in more detail in the context of specific research approaches in the following chapters, but broadly speaking designs that have a quantitative orientation tend to work with larger sample sizes than those with a qualitative orientation. The reason for this comes back to the purpose of the research in the first instance. If you were undertaking a qualitative study designed to identify how people feel about having a leg amputated you might suggest that the purpose of this study was to gain insight into the feelings that people have in order to increase your sensitivity when caring for people with this problem. This being the case, it is sufficient for you to approach a small number of people and spend some time with them exploring in depth what they feel. The emphasis on sample selection is on identifying a group of respondents who have the 'experience' of the phenomenon being studied.

However, if in contrast you were a scientist developing a new sun-tan lotion it would not be sufficient to test it on a small number of people. What you would want to know is whether your product will be effective for the general population. Selecting a few people might illustrate a good result but might fail to indicate possible side effects, such as skin rashes, that may occur as a result of the product if it was used by a greater number. Therefore, in quantitative research studies, emphasis is placed on the way in which samples are selected to ensure that they are *representative* of the population as a whole. Depending on the target populations this might involve the selection of large numbers or at least a selection of sufficient numbers to enable statistical tests to be used to indicate whether the results of the study can be accredited to the product under review; in this case, sun-tan cream.

The key factor to consider when determining the population to be studied is the nature of the research design. If the purpose of the study is to get results that can be generalised across the population being studied then the researcher must identify a *random sample*. This means that every member of the population being studied has an equal chance of being selected for the sample and is a technique used to select samples from a population in such as way as to avoid the presence of bias in the sample selection. Thus a random sample is said to be a true representation of a given population.

For example, if the researcher wanted to do a study of midwifery practice throughout the country he or she would need to ensure that all practising midwives had an equal opportunity of being involved in the research. This could be a mammoth task as there are many thousands of midwives and so the researcher may attempt to become more specific in defining the population by deciding, for example, to focus on midwives based in hospital units as this is where most deliveries take place. The group is still large so a further exclusion may be done by making the focus of the study all those midwives who have been practising in their field for five years or more and so may be considered 'expert'. The researcher may also consider it important to include 'only those midwives who work full time and so on. These factors or variables might impact on the outcome of the research and may be described as *confounding variables*. A confounding variable is a variable that varies systematically with the variables being studied and so provides an alternative explanation for any effects. So, for example, whether midwives work full or part time is an important point as the views of the two groups may be different. Failure to recognise this introduces a source of *error* in the research, that is the results may be distorted. If potential errors are recognised and predictable they are referred to as *constant errors*; if they are not predictable they are described as *random errors*. We will return to this issue in the context of statistical testing in Chapter 10.

The nature of the research being planned will determine the extent to which the researcher specifies the criteria for sample selection. Commonly researchers will indicate inclusion and exclusion criteria when determining their sample. As you can see from this the sample above is clearly focusing on hospital-based midwifery practices drawing on experienced midwives who are working full time. Exclusion criteria in this case would be those midwives working in the community, having less experience or working part time.

The next problem would be how to identify this potential sample group. The researcher could approach the Royal College of Midwives and ask for a list of practising midwives but it is unlikely that the College would be able to help, mainly because of confidentiality – professional organisations keep lists for their own records, they are not records kept for public access regardless of the purpose for requesting them. Perhaps another option would be to identify all hospital units and approach the managers of that unit and ask if they would be willing to help in the project. The same issues of confidentiality would apply here but at least it would be possible to approach a number of unnamed midwives and ask for co-operation. It would depend on the perceived value of the research from the managers' perspective as to whether they would be willing to help out or not. They may be willing but unable to do so as the staff may already be involved in another research study or some similar project.

The researcher will still be left with a large population from which to select a sample for this study. In so doing he or she may choose to undertake a process of *probability sampling* which implies using random sampling procedures. For example the potential sample of midwives may run into many thousands, and to involve so many people in a research project may, for this researcher, be unrealistic. So the next step would be to select a *random sample* which will give a true representation of the whole population of midwives. This could be done very simply by taking the whole list of practising midwives who have been practising for five years of more and working full time in hospital practice and selecting names of potential participants 'out of a hat'. Alternatively the researcher may allocate each midwife on the list a number and use a random sample table, available in many statistical books. Details and instructions on how to use these tables are generally included in texts on statistics.

As the example above indicates, choosing a true random sample is possible but quite complex in health care research. There are some ways in which this approach is modified to give the research a little more control over the sample mix. For example a *stratified random sample* would enable the researcher to select people from two or more strata of the population independently, for example, junior and senior practitioners. The important point to remember is that random sampling is the most reliable way of ensuring that you get a representative view from the population you will be studying. Because of this, in quantitative research, if you are unable to get a random sample there will be some implications if you wanted to undertake statistical testing of data in some quantitative research designs (see Chapter 10).

As the process of selecting a random sample can be very unwieldy other approaches may be used, sometimes referred to as *non-probability sampling*. It is not uncommon for researchers to choose a *sample of convenience*: a sample selected on the basis of convenience for the researcher in situations where it is not possible to get a random sample. For example, the researcher in the midwifery study above may decide to focus the study on midwives working in two or three hospitals seen to be typical of hospitals of that type. Rigorous criteria could be used in selecting centres in an attempt to avoid introducing *bias* into the study by weak sampling techniques, and the limitations in sampling are noted in the final report of the study. This is important, for factors such as geographical location can make a difference – there may be quite a different attitude, say, between people living and working in inner city hospitals in London and those working in a more rural hospital in the north for example.

To try to minimise the risk of bias if using a sample of convenience the researcher may still employ the principles of random sampling in determining which members of a given population will be studied. So, out of a group of 100 midwives chosen as a sample of convenience for the study, the researcher may select a percentage of these using random sampling techniques, as the final sample for the research.

It should be noted that although the results from such small-scale studies have only limited scope in terms of generalising findings to all situations, results from one small study may, however, lend support to the findings of another similar study. Together these studies can be used to direct changes in practice if this is appropriate. For this reason there is value in replicating research studies in health care research as indicated earlier.

In qualitative research designs there are some other considerations that will be discussed in the context of this approach in Chapter 7.

Other factors affecting sampling

There are other issues that the researcher must consider when determining his or her sample for a study. Organisational factors may mitigate against the researcher wishing to do a study of a given population. For example, the researcher may have conceived a study which incorporates distributing questionnaires to third year students on health care programmes working in general hospital wards on a given day. It is quite feasible that the researcher's plan and the organisation's plan do not coincide for, on the chosen day, all third year students in that hospital are unavailable! Obviously careful planning could help avoid this situation happening, but this example highlights how the potential for change within organisations have an impact on a proposed study.

A second point in relation to this is that geographical factors may also play a part in determining suitable samples. The nurse who decides to investigate the 'public image of nurses' may get totally different responses from a selection of people going in and out of hospital waiting areas and a random sample of people shopping in the high street on a Saturday afternoon. The implications are that this has introduced bias into the study.

Awareness of the potential problem of introducing bias into a study is important. For example if undertaking a study of patients' reactions to their hospital experience a researcher may find that a group of patients in hospital may give a different response from a group of people who have been discharged from hospital and had time to ponder on their experience. Both views need to be considered in studies of this nature, as obviously location and potential vulnerability can make a difference to the way in which patients may respond.

Pilot study

A pilot study is seen as a small-scale 'test' of the research design of a proposed study and is a useful exercise before embarking on the main project. The purpose of the pilot study is to identify any potential weaknesses in the design of the study. For the researcher using qualitative approaches this gives an opportunity to test the proposed techniques of data collection. The same is true for the researcher undertaking a quantitatively orientated study, although in this case there will be an added dimension of using the piloting stage to develop and test the research instruments (see Chapter 9). As it is a test of the main study it is important that respondents in the pilot study reflect, as near as possible, the sample of people that will be the population of the main study.

There are several factors that will contribute towards the decision to undertake a pilot study. The first of these may be the research design itself: some methods of enquiry do not lend themselves to a 'trial run'. The size of the research project is another factor to consider. Some practitioners feel that there is little point in doing a pilot study if their proposed research is on a very small scale. This may occur, for example, if undertaking a project as part of an undergraduate programme where the emphasis is on learning about research design. For this group it is still advisable that some sort of *pre-test* is undertaken to test the validity of any research instruments used. A 'pre-test' is seen as an opportunity to test research instruments rather than a replication of the proposed study as in the pilot study. (NB See also Chapter 8 regarding the use of the term pre-test in experimental design as this may cause confusion. In experimental design the pre-test is an integral part of the study.) Following a pilot study the researcher may, if it is seen necessary, modify the research tools before proceeding with the main study.

Data analysis

The researcher should consider how information, or data, collected should be analysed *in the design stage of the research study*. As with all aspects of research, careful planning in relation to this can help avoid the pitfall of collecting a lot of information and not being sure what to do with it once it has been obtained. In research reports the analysis of data should be clear, concise and reflect a fair picture of what was found in the course of the study. Methods of analysing and presenting data in qualitative and quantitative research designs are explored in Chapter 10.

Ethical approval

In Chapter 4 the ethical dilemmas in research were discussed and so will not be repeated here except to emphasise that any potential ethical dilemmas need to be clarified at the outset and appropriate permission to undertake the work granted. As noted in Chapter 4 the policies in some districts and health care trusts vary, and you may be required to submit only those requiring access to patients and clients whilst others may ask you to submit all proposed research studies to the ethical committees.

Access

The need to obtain permission to access potential research subjects was discussed in Chapter 4. Access differs from ethical approval as it indicates that you have sought permission through the appropriate management structure to access your client group. Getting permission to proceed on ethical grounds does not mean you have permission to access the potential subjects. For example, if you wished to access a group of schoolchildren to explore their knowledge of health promotion activities you might have ethical approval to proceed but you would still need to approach the headteacher of the school and possibly the board of governors to be allowed to proceed. In health care it can be more complex as, depending on the managerial structure, you may need to seek permission through both professional and organisational channels. Managers will want to know how you are going to ensure the confidentiality of the staff and patients involved in the study and what you are going to do with the results. It is good practice to offer to feed the research results back to the research site.

The research report

At the end of the research study the researcher must write a full report of the work and findings. Failure to do so implies that he or she need not have done the research in the first place as the overall purpose of research is to develop the knowledge in the area of study. In concluding their work many researchers will make recommendations for action based on their findings. The reader of research reports should be alert to the style of presentation of information and make particular note as to whether the information in the final report matches the findings noted earlier in the study. In writing the report the researcher should obviously give an unbiased account of the study and the interpretation of the findings. As writing skills are seen to be a very important aspect of research this topic is discussed in more detail in Chapter 11.

Disseminating research activity

Writing a research report is not the final step. If you were to complete a research project and simply leave it sitting on a shelf, then the same principle of 'why did you bother?' applies. So the final stage of a research project is the dissemination of findings. This is increasingly important in the context of present-day research and development strategies and is discussed in more detail in Chapter 12.

ACTIVITY _____

- Select several research reports from your own professional journals.
- Refer to Table 6.1 to remind yourself of the difference you might expect between qualitative and quantitative research.
- Answer the following questions in relation to each article:

    Is the research problem defined?
    Is there a comprehensive literature review?
    Is the research design clear?

Are the techniques of data collection stated?
Are the population and sample selection defined?
Was a pilot study completed?
How were the data analysed?
Were any potential ethical dilemmas noted and ethical approval sought?
Was the means of gaining access to the research site discussed?
Is the research report easy to read and understand?
Has the researcher indicated any efforts to disseminate the findings to clinical practice?

Summary

This chapter has given an outline of the research process following the format noted in Table 6.1. In highlighting the stages of the research process this chapter also gives a source of reference for readers who want to learn how to read research reports critically as the topic areas discussed give a broad outline on which to develop this skill, as indicated in the activity above.

Further reading

Abbott, P. and Sapsford, R. (1992) *Research into Practice. A Reader for Nurses and the Caring Professions*, Open University Press, Buckingham.

Bell, J. (1993) *Doing Your Research Project? A Guide for First Time Researchers in Education and the Social Sciences*, Open University Press, Buckingham.

Berger, R.M. and Patchup, M.A. (1988) *Planning for Research. A Guide for the Helping Professions*, Sage, London.

Brockopp, D.Y. and Hastings-Tolsma, M.T. (1995) *Fundamentals of Nursing Research*, 2nd edn, Jones & Bartlett, Boston.

Carnwell, R. (1997) *Evaluative Research Methodology in Nursing and Health Care*, Open Learning Foundation/Churchill Livingstone, Edinburgh.

Carr, L.T. (1994) 'The strengths and weaknesses of quantitative and qualitative research: what method for nursing?', *Journal of Advanced Nursing*, vol. 20, no. 4, pp. 716–721.

Chapman, J. (1991) 'Research – What it is and what it is not', in Perry, A. and Jolley, M., *Nursing – A Knowledge Base for Practice*, Edward Arnold, London, Ch. 2.

Clamp, C. (1994) *Resources for Nursing Research: An Annotated Bibliography*, 2nd edn, Library Association, London.

Clifford, C., Carnwell, R. and Harkin, L. (1996) *Research Methodology in Nursing and Health Care*, Open Learning Foundation/Churchill Livingstone, Edinburgh.

Cormack, D.F.S. (1991) *The Research Process in Nursing*, 2nd edn, Blackwell Scientific Publications, Oxford.

Corner, J. (1991) 'In search of more complete answers to research questions. Quantitative vs qualitative research methods: is there a way forward?', *Journal of Advanced Nursing*, vol. 16, pp. 718–727.

Holter, I.M. and Schwartz-Barcott, D. (1993) 'Action research: what is it? How has it been used and how can it be used in nursing?', *Journal of Advanced Nursing*, vol. 18, no. 2, pp. 298–304.

Phillips, C., Palfrey, C. and Thomas, P. (1994) *Evaluating Health and Social Care*, Macmillan, London.

Sapsford, R. and Abbott, P. (1992) *Research Methods for Nurses and the Caring Professions*, Open University Press, Buckingham.

Stake, R.E. (1995) *The Art of Case Study Research*, Sage, London.

You are also referred to the journal: 'Action Research', *Nurse Research*, vol. 2, no. 3, March (1995).

7   Research designs using qualitative approaches

Qualitative research fits into the category of descriptive research design in that the focus is on finding out what is happening in a given situation rather than trying to explain relationships or cause and effect. However, this can sometimes cause confusion to newcomers to research because descriptive designs may also be used in a quantitative way such as in the use of surveys in which data can be analysed numerically. When using a descriptive research design to collect quantifiable data the researcher is looking for trends in larger numbers of respondents. This contrasts with the search for 'depth of understanding' or meaning found in descriptive designs used to collect non-numeric or 'qualitative' data. It has been noted throughout this text that the approach to research depends on the question you are asking. If your question was orientated towards the individual perspective in asking questions such as 'what does this mean?' or 'how does it feel?' you would be more likely to develop a research design that collects qualitative data.

In this chapter we will consider some of the approaches that are categorised as qualitative research design and will consider the following:

1. The features of qualitative research.
2. Planning for qualitative research studies.
3. Approaches to qualitative research.

Features of qualitative research

The underlying principle of all qualitative research is that it is descriptive in nature. Researchers completing qualitative research studies will seek to 'tell it how it is' rather than attempt to identify trends or find relationships in the data, such as you might find in research designs using quantitative approaches.

Qualitative research is characterised by three features. The first is that qualitative research design is at the *inductive* end of the knowledge development continuum. If you refer back to Chapter 5 you will note that knowledge development was described at several levels, ranging from identification of concepts using inductive approaches to proposing and testing relationships between them which use deductive approaches.

The focus of qualitative research is commonly about unearthing new knowledge or getting new insights and so is at the inductive end of knowledge development.

The second feature of qualitative research design is that the research is conducted in such a way as to consider the *emic* perspective, that is from the perspective of the individual participants being studied. This is another feature that makes the qualitative approach distinct from quantitative research designs which commonly look for patterns or trends in the larger population in which the 'etic' perspective dominates (i.e. the perspective of the researcher or outsider).

Linked to this, qualitative researchers claim their approaches are more *holistic*. The focus on the individual includes consideration of the context in which the research takes place. The emphasis here is on the 'real world' and the researcher endeavours to collect data in the context of everyday life in which the normal range of life experiences are taken into account. Researchers using a qualitative approach commonly refer to collecting data 'in the field', which they use to mean the natural setting in which the research occurs. Furthermore, the qualitative researcher places emphasis on the values held by the individual, a factor that is often overlooked in quantitative research design. For example, with experimental research designs the researcher endeavours to control and manipulate the 'real world' by excluding certain variables from the study to measure specific effects of variables identified. This leads to accusations of 'context stripping' – taking aspects of human behaviour out of the context in which they occur. Qualitative researchers seek to collect data in the 'real world' and so do not change the context.

In summary it can be seen that the approaches to research classified under the qualitative umbrella are said to be inductive, developing knowledge from the emic perspective and holistic. This is not an exclusive list of features of qualitative research design but is indicative of the broad principles of qualitative design.

As you will see later, there are different theoretical influences that shape the way qualitative research designs are developed and will impact on the way in which the research is developed. There are an increasing number of texts being produced for the health and social care readership extolling the values of different approaches to qualitative research design. Such claims can serve to confuse unless you have a broad insight into the differing influences that may affect the research design chosen for qualitative work, and so you need to consider this in the context of planning for qualitative research.

Planning for qualitative research

As noted in the last chapter the starting point when planning for a research study is to determine the problem area and, from this, the *questions* you want answered. This will help establish the approach that would be appropriate to adopt. Commonly in qualitative research designs the research question provides the main focus for the study. This contrasts with quantitative designs which, as you will see, commonly develop the research question into more specific frameworks using aims, objectives and hypotheses for experimental designs.

The next point is to consider the use of *literature*. As you will see below, the approach to the literature in qualitative research designs varies depending on the overall approach to the study. In some instances you may choose to undertake a qualitative research study because, in the course of your literature review, you have found there is very limited information available on your chosen topic. This indicates a need to identify some of the key concepts before moving on to a different level of knowledge development (see Chapter 5). Alternatively you might have found a lot of literature on the topic but noted that all the research so far had been undertaken in a highly structured quantitative manner with little note taken of the origins of concepts used – so you might set out to challenge some assumptions in various theories presented by exploring the subject from a qualitative perspective.

Some qualitative approaches to research involve deferring the literature review until you have developed the research design a little more to try to keep your mind 'empty' of existing thoughts on the topic and consequently receptive to new ideas. An example of this is the grounded theory approach we will discuss below. Although this might be an ideal in terms of research design, it is quite difficult to do in health care research directed at practical issues since the literature is used to justify why a given study is important. You may be able to start with an 'empty slate' if you are undertaking a project for a degree, for example, and your supervisors advise you to do this. However, if you want to submit a proposal for funds to support your research there are very few funding organisations which accept a proposal with a justification not supported by existing literature. Consequently, it may be necessary to complete this in the early stages of a study before applying for funds.

Approaches to qualitative research design

The next step to consider is the approach you might take to the research design. If you refer to Figure 7.1 you will see that under the heading of qualitative research four types of qualitative research have been identified:

1. Descriptive.
2. Ethnography.
3. Phenomenology.
4. Grounded theory.

Each of these will be discussed further below.

The descriptive approach to qualitative research

It has been suggested earlier that all qualitative research will be, by definition, descriptive in that no attempt is made to manipulate the data or the situation being observed, to look for relationships or cause and effect. In identifying a category as 'descriptive research' it should be noted that this is a term used in both qualitative and quantitative research design. In both instances it is used to define an approach

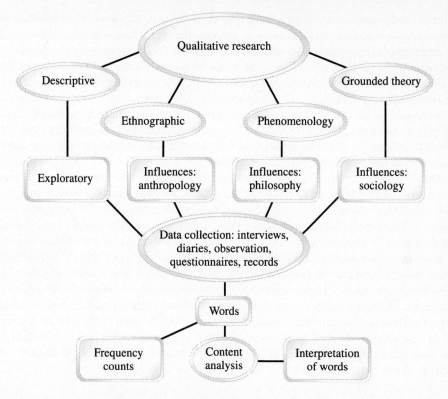

Figure 7.1 Overview of qualitative research design.

to research which simply reports on what is observed, that is it describes the existing situation. The distinction between both approaches is that descriptive approaches used in qualitative research will collect data in words, whilst descriptive approaches in quantitative research studies facilitate numerical analysis of data using descriptive statistics. We will return to this in the next chapter.

The descriptive approach to qualitative research is useful when researchers want to undertake a study which utilises the principles of qualitative research design to explore situations but do not identify a clear theoretical focus found in other approaches to qualitative research. Sometimes the word 'exploratory' is used to describe this approach.

To illustrate the use of a descriptive approach to qualitative design let us consider a simple example of a health care worker who wants to undertake a study in his or her own clinical area to find out how people with rheumatoid arthritis feel about the disabilities that disease causes. To answer this question the researcher decides to explore this issue further by undertaking a qualitative study and interviewing some people with arthritis about their feelings. The purpose of this would be to give an account of the feelings this group has about the disease. This interview might consist of some open questions asking people how they feel, what specific problems they feel they have, any strategies they use to overcome their problems and any other aspects of their disease they might like to discuss and so on. In giving an account of the data collected from the interviews the researcher may summarise the main themes that emerge in the data and report that – in other words describing what they observe.

Information gathered by descriptive qualitative approaches such as this can be used at several levels. At one level it can serve to give the researcher greater insight in the nature of the problems his or her clients may have. If the researcher then writes this project into a research report (see Chapter 11) that knowledge may be shared with colleagues and help to increase their insight also.

Data collected from descriptive studies such as this that explore a particular phenomenon can be used to develop further enquiry. The researcher may find that the interviews have raised a number of issues about the problems people with rheumatoid arthritis face and so they may decide to use the data they have collected to develop a further research study. For example the data may be used to develop a more structured questionnaire designed to ask a larger sample of people with rheumatoid arthritis how they feel about their disease. As you will see in Chapter 9 it is not uncommon for researchers to use quotes raised by people in the interview stage of a study to structure a more detailed questionnaire survey. However, it should be noted that this would only be appropriate if this was part of the overall research design in which a researcher stated at the outset that this was how the data were to be used. This will be discussed further in the context of data analysis in Chapter 10.

The ethnographic approach to qualitative research

One approach widely adopted by qualitative researchers is ethnography. Ethnography is the study of cultures in which researchers seek to describe and explain the cultures observed. Researchers using an ethnographic approach are doing so using the theoretical influences developed in anthropology in which the focus of the study is on 'culture' or a group of individuals in their normal habitat.

The opportunities to study cultures in health care are endless and, if you wanted to use this approach, the first step would be to decide which 'culture' you wish to study. The 'culture' you choose to study may be a staff culture, a patient or client culture, or a specific culture in society. For example, if studying a staff culture you may wish to describe and explain the 'culture' of the primary health care team. If studying a 'client culture' you may wish to explore the culture experienced by a client in a long-term care ward. If studying a specific culture in society you might wish to understand the drug-taking culture or the adolescent culture and so on.

The key features in the ethnographic approach lie in the ability of the researcher to 'get inside' the culture and to understand that culture from the point of view of the participants. From this perspective the term 'going native' has been coined to describe the process that researchers may go through to explore, describe and analyse the culture being studied. The suggestion here is that the more fully the researcher absorbs the culture, the more he or she will understand the values and beliefs of the people in that culture.

There is thus a need to consider the best ways to collect data to understand the values of the people in the culture. In ethnographic research this will include observation, asking questions through interviews and, in some instances, using more structured approaches, for example questionnaires. In addition to this the researcher may access records, historical documents, diaries and other forms of data to build a complete 'picture' of the culture being studied. So, if the researcher was planning to examine the culture of the client in the long-term care ward for example, he or she would spend long periods of time in that ward, observe what was going on and interview the range of people involved in the ward. This might include the patients/clients, their relatives, the nurses, physiotherapists, occupational therapists, speech therapists, social workers, dieticians, chaplain, etc. In addition the researcher might draw on people's experiences through a review of documentation pertaining to the development of the ward and, if available, might use personal records, diaries, etc. An important point in the data collection is that the researcher must attempt to establish the validity of the data. This can be done by returning ideas and views to the participants and asking for their opinions (see Chapter 10).

So, it can be seen that ethnography involves studying people in their natural environment with the researcher being intimately involved in the data collection process. To understand what is happening in that culture the researcher will draw on numerous sources of data, probably over a long time period. The anthropologists build up the picture of what is happening in a culture by extensive '*field*' work, that is collecting data in the field – the natural habitat of the people being studied. The context for the field work is an important point and the researcher needs to relate the study to current and future events. For example, an exploration in a long-term care ward in the 1990s must be considered in the context of changing patterns of care considering the importance of care in the community, as this has had a major impact on institutional care.

As this approach draws on a wide range of skill of data collection it needs to be used very cautiously by the newcomer to research who is only just developing these skills. Moreover, as was noted in Chapter 4 the issue of time available to undertake a given project can influence the research design and it may be that although you have a preference for undertaking an ethnographic study, the time available to you to develop one is not available. Consequently, researchers who are faced with constraints of this nature may proceed with developing research studies from an ethnographic perspective at the outset, note the aim of the study is to understand the culture but acknowledge the limitations that may impact on the design adopted. In other words the research can be influenced by the ethnographic perspective even though not constituting a full-blown ethnographic study.

The phenomenological approach to qualitative research

The phenomenological approach to qualitative research endeavours to understand the subjective viewpoint of the individuals being studied. The source of knowledge influencing this approach can be closely related to philosophical reasoning (see Chapter 5). The focus of the research contrasts with the study of groups in a given culture in ethnography and is clearly directed towards the subjective view of the individual being studied.

The phenomenological approach can be quite a complex process as it relies on the researcher's skill in drawing information and interpreting data rather than a structured approach that will tell you 'how to do phenomenology'. Researchers try to understand the subjective view of the individual but, in so doing, recognise that that subjectivity is interpreted by the researchers themselves.

To develop this approach there is a need to consider how best to understand the subjective meaning to the individual. This is a useful starting point, for it prompts the researcher towards deciding the appropriate techniques of data collection. You cannot find out how someone feels if you 'put the words in their mouths' in the form of a structured questionnaire, therefore you discard that option. You might be able to gain insight into feeling by reading written records such as diaries and it may be that the best way in which you might answer this is to talk to people. Now as the researcher is trying to understand how people feel about something and is seeking to interpret that data he or she would need to go back to the respondent to check their interpretation. Consequently, the technique used in phenomenology research is largely interviews. The researcher will commonly return to the interviewee on more than one occasion to discuss the interpretation, to check whether the respondents views are being appropriately illustrated and so on. This is important in determining the validity of the study.

Other techniques of data collection can be considered with caution. For example, you cannot understand how people feel about things by watching them, therefore any use of observation techniques of data collection must be used with caution. If observation techniques are used they are more likely to involve participant observation which involves the researcher working alongside the person being observed. This, with observing, enables the researcher to participate in discussion in the course of activities as a technique of data collection.

Throughout phenomenological studies the emphasis is on the individual's perspective as seen through the eyes of the researcher. Sampling techniques are designed to reflect the phenomenon being studied so, for example, a researcher who wants to undertake a phenomenological study of nurses working in an acute hospital would focus purposefully on nurses working in acute hospitals when selecting a sample.

Some texts will explain how phenomenological researchers 'bracket' their own experiences in an endeavour to ensure they do not put too much of their views into the data analysis. Although the researchers are an active participant in the research process, they study the phenomenon from the perspective of the respondent with the emphasis on the experience from the respondent's viewpoint. Clearly this is a very inductive approach.

The grounded theory approach and qualitative research

The grounded theory approach has been developed from the social sciences as a means of developing a theory that is 'grounded in reality' about the social world.

The starting point would be a descriptor of the social situation being observed and, through the study, the researcher attempts to develop a theory about the social situation based on a combination of data collected by a range of techniques and literature review. An influence in this is the concept of 'symbolic interaction' which focuses on how individuals relate to situations observed. In this approach the literature is used as the study progresses to help inform and develop the emerging theory.

Although generally discussed in the context of qualitative research design some aspects of grounded theory are clearly influenced by the techniques used in quantitative research. For example, the rigorous approach to data analysis which demands a clear explanation of the procedure followed shows similar characteristics to the models of data analysis adopted in quantitative approaches and thus leads to claims that grounded theory is a more 'scientific approach' than other qualitative methods. Also, grounded theory differs from the other approaches outlined above in that, from the outset, the researcher sets out to use both qualitative and quantitative approaches to data collection to develop a theory from the emergent data. Consequently both inductive and deductive approaches are used with the research design as the researcher develops ideas from data generated inductively and then tests out the ideas deductively. As emergent theory is tested it may lead the researcher back to the inductive mode to explore new ideas that have emerged.

To do this grounded theory is characterised by a prescriptive approach to data analysis which involves the researcher in constant comparison of data as they emerge, and a consequent search for 'alternative cases' that may challenge the emergent theory. This constant comparison is designed to help refine and so maximise the credibility of the theory that emerges.

To this end sampling is directed at identifying an initial sample to help clarify the area of study and, thereafter, to draw on sampling groups that may inform the developing theory; hence the term *theoretical sampling* is used. The developing theory guides the data that need to be collected and helps refine the focus of the data collection. The researcher needs to be constantly alert to the data collected – theoretical sensitivity. To help this, the way in which data are analysed is closely prescribed for the grounded theories and involves a process of coding that is described in a step by step process in the texts on its topic.

The subject of grounded theory can sound rather complex when overviews such as this are offered. Consequently any reader interested in developing this approach is recommended to the further reading at the end of the chapter.

Data collection in qualitative research

The techniques of data collection will be reviewed in Chapter 9. However, it should be noted at this stage that the techniques of data collection used in research are, in principle, the same for both qualitative and quantitative research approaches. They include the use of questionnaires, interviews, observation, access to records, diaries and so on. However, the difference between the approaches lies in the *structure* of the instruments used and, arising from this, the type of data collected. In qualitative research, for example, questionnaires or interviews would include *open questions* designed to let respondents answer in their own words. The same principle applies to using observation as a means of collecting data. In qualitative research the observer would keep open *field notes*, that is the notes kept when undertaking an observation study 'in the field' (i.e. the natural setting). These ways of using the research tools can be contrasted with quantitative research in which a highly structured questionnaire and observation tools would be used which limit respondents to a fixed range of responses.

Sampling techniques in qualitative design

The nature of the sample that is used in qualitative research design is clearly directed to the question being asked and the underlying principles of the research. The first point to remember is that qualitative researchers are trying to understand the situation they are observing. As the researcher focuses on the meaning of a given situation he or she is not generally worried about whether what is being observed can be applied to a whole population. Thus, unlike the quantitatively orientated researcher, the emphasis in sample selection in qualitative research design is generally on *small*, clearly identified sample groups commonly using a *sample of convenience*, that is a sample that is readily accessible to the researcher.

To some extent, at a practical level, the nature of sampling in qualitative research design is determined by the nature of data collection. If a researcher wanted to spend thirty or forty minutes interviewing people to ask them 'How do you feel about your life?' it would not be a good idea to approach hundreds of people for interview. First this would involve many hours of interviewing, and secondly it would involve many more hours of analysing the data. This is quite a time-consuming exercise in qualitative research. As you will see in Chapter 8 this contrasts quite markedly with quantitative research approaches where the emphasis is often on getting representative samples of the population.

So, for example, if a health care researcher wanted to do a study about quality of life for people with chronic pain, they would purposefully select their sample from people known to have chronic pain. Thus one type of sampling in qualitative research design is described as *purposeful sampling* in which the researcher goes out to collect data purposefully from the respondent. As indicated above, different terms may be used by different researchers to give focus to their sampling technique. So, as noted, the grounded theorist would use the term *theoretical sampling* to indicate the driving force in sample selection as that of the emergent theory.

Sometimes the qualitative researcher may select the sample in an opportunistic way. For example, if a health care researcher was undertaking a study of people with chronic pain and a person with this problem was identified to them by their colleagues in day-to-day practice, they might approach that person and ask if he or she would be willing to be involved in the study (adhering to the agreed ethical principles of the research design). This is known as *opportunistic sampling*. Another approach that is sometimes used in qualitative research is *snowball sampling* techniques. Here the

researcher identifies the sample by cascading from one research subject to another –
for example if talking to the person with chronic pain the researcher might ask the
respondent if they know anyone else with the same problem who might be willing
to talk to them.

Data analysis in qualitative design

As you can see in Figure 7.1 qualitative research designs involve collecting non-
numerical data. The words may be the result of using open questions and interviews
or, by a researcher making notes as part of the field work in a study involving
observation. Other forms of data in words can be generated by referring to records
or diaries that contribute to the phenomenon being studied. For example the *historical
research* will use qualitative research methods to help explore and analyse past events.

The process of data analysis commonly used in qualitative researcher design is
described as *content analysis*. This is discussed in more detail in Chapter 10. You will
see that in Figure 7.1 there is an indication that in some instances the process of
content analysis may lead to some level of counting the data frequency. This issue
will be discussed further in Chapter 10.

ACTIVITY _____

- Consider an area of your work in which a qualitative study could be
  carried out.
- State what type of qualitative study you would use for your example.
- How would you collect the data for your study?
- What do you think might be the strengths and limitations of the approach
  you have chosen?

Summary

In this chapter a broad overview of qualitative approaches to research has been
presented. The features of qualitative research have been identified and the issue you
might need to consider when planning a qualitative research study considered. Several
different approaches to the research design have been outlined. Any reader intending
to utilise one of these approaches is advised to follow up the further reading at the
end of the chapter, particularly those texts that give a specific instruction as to how
to approach these techniques.

Further reading

Chenitz, W.C. and Swanson, J.M. (1986) *From Practice to Grounded Theory: Qualitative Research
in Nursing*, Addison-Wesley, Menlo Park, California.

Clarke, E. (1991) *Research Awareness Module 7 The Ethnographic Perspective*, Distance Learning Centre, South Bank Polytechnic (South Bank University), London.

Clarke, L. (1992) 'Qualitative research: meaning and language', *Journal of Advanced Nursing*, vol. 17, pp. 243–252.

Clifford, C. (1997) *Qualitative Research Methodology in Nursing and Health Care*, Open Learning Foundation/Churchill Livingstone, Edinburgh.

Denzin, N.K. and Lincoln, Y.S. (1994) *Handbook of Qualitative Research*, Sage, London.

Field, P.A. and Morse, J. (1996) *Nursing Research: The Application of Qualitative Approaches*, Chapman & Hall, London.

Holloway, I. and Wheeler, S. (1996) *Qualitative Research for Nurses*, Blackwell Scientific, Oxford.

Holstein, J.A. and Gubrian, J.F. (1994) 'Phenomenology, ethnomethodology and interpretative practice', in Denzin, N.K. and Lincoln, Y.S., *Handbook of Qualitative Research*, Sage, London, Ch. 16.

Leininger, M.M. (Ed.) (1985) *Qualitative Research Methods in Nursing*, Grune & Stratton, Orlando, FL.

Marchus, G.E. (1994) 'What comes (just) after "Post"? The case of ethnography', in Denzin, N.K. and Lincoln, Y.S., *Handbook of Qualitative Research*, Sage, London, Ch. 35.

Marshall, C. and Rossman, G.B. (1989) *Designing Qualitative Research*, Sage, London.

Miles, M.B. and Hubermans, A.M. (1994) *Qualitative Data Analysis*, Sage, London.

Morse, J.M. (Ed.) (1991) *Qualitative Nursing Research – A Contemporary Dialogue*, Sage, London.

Morse, J.M. (Ed.) (1994) *Critical Issues in Qualitative Research*, Sage, London.

Moustakis, C. (1994) *Phenomenological Research Methods*, Sage, London.

Munhall, P.L. and Oiler, C.J. (1986) *Nursing Research: A Qualitative Perspective*, Appleton Century Crofts, Connecticut.

Strauss, A. and Corbin, J. (1990) *Basics of Qualitative Research*, Sage, London.

Strauss, A. and Corbin, J. (1994) 'Grounded theory methodology: An overview', in Denzin, N.K. and Lincoln, Y.S., *Handbook of Qualitative Research*, Sage, London, Ch. 17.

Taylor, B.J. (1994) *Being Human: Ordinariness in Nursing*, Churchill Livingstone, Edinburgh.

You are also referred to the following journals: *Qualitative Health Research*, published monthly, and 'Ethnography and Phenomenology', *Nurse Researcher*, vol. 2, no. 2, December (1995).

8   Research designs using quantitative approaches

In earlier chapters it has been noted that when planning the research design for a study a number of different approaches are classed under the quantitative research umbrella. These range from descriptive through to experimental research design as indicated in Figure 8.1. It is on this range of approaches that this chapter will focus and we will consider the following:

1. Descriptive research designs in quantitative research.
2. Correlational research designs.
3. Experimental research design.
4. Quasi-experimental research designs.

Each of these approaches serves a different purpose and addresses different aspects of the research process slightly differently as outlined in Figure 8.2 which links the stages of the research process with the overall research design.

Descriptive research designs in quantitative research

It was noted in Chapter 6 that when considering research from a descriptive perspective we could include both qualitative and quantitative aspects in the research design. As indicated in the last chapter qualitative research is always descriptive but you can also develop descriptive studies that have a clear quantitative orientation. In this

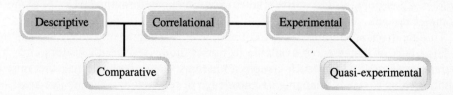

Figure 8.1 Research designs using quantitative approaches to data collection and analysis.

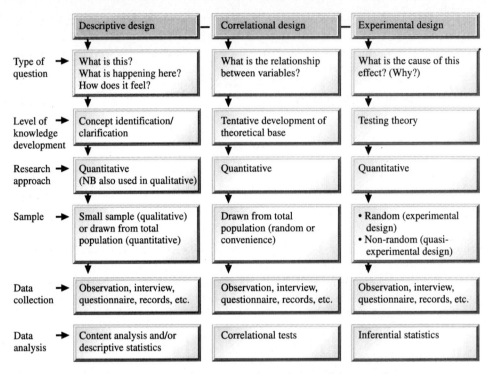

Figure 8.2 Research designs using quantitative approaches and stages of the research process.

chapter we will focus on the quantitative dimension of descriptive research. As noted in Chapter 6, it is important to recognise that it is not uncommon for both quantitative and qualitative dimensions to be included in a single study.

Descriptive research, as the name implies, is the kind of research that 'describes' what is happening in a given situation. This type of research may also be referred to as *non-experimental* research, a term commonly used to indicate that it does not have the features of experimental research design that we will discuss below. Another term used by researchers beginning to explore some phenomenon is *exploratory research*. This may also be associated with descriptive research as it commonly seeks to describe what is seen in a given situation. The value of this approach is that it frequently opens our eyes to what is happening around us. Moreover, as we will see later, it is important that base line information is accurate before undertaking more complex studies. Consequently, descriptive studies may sometimes form the first stage of more complex designs.

To date descriptive approaches to quantitative research have tended to make up a large part of the research available to nurses, midwives, health visitors and the paramedical professions (such as physiotherapists and occupational therapists), although this is slowly changing as knowledge of research and the subject areas of professional practice increases. There are perhaps two reasons for this. The first is that in any discipline starting out in research there may be a limited knowledge base from which to develop more complex studies. The first issue to be considered in any research should be clarification of what is actually happening in a given situation. Building on this, and perhaps another reason that descriptive research designs are so popular, is that for the newcomer to research descriptive designs may not be perceived as being as complex as the other approaches we will be discussing below. This may be an important consideration to students undertaking research projects in a limited time period. However, at a more philosophical level it was noted in earlier chapters that when making decisions about what type of research to do the researcher needs to consider the research questions and purpose of the research.

The starting point for a quantitative descriptive research design is to state the research *aims and objectives* clearly. This sets the framework for the study and gives the building block from which the research can be developed. Generally speaking one overall aim and four or five objectives arising from this are sufficient for most descriptive research studies. So, the researcher might set their aims and objectives as indicated below:

AIM _____

To identify the factors influencing communication amongst members of the multi-disciplinary health care team.

Objectives: To survey all members of the multi-disciplinary team to determine their:

- views on written communication;
- views on verbal communication;
- perceptions of impediments to communication;
- perceptions of factors that enhance good communication.

The aims and objectives give a focus to this study and set the parameters to the questions that will be asked as the study is developed. Subsumed under the overall aim or 'main idea' are a range of variables that are seen to impact on the issue of multi-disciplinary communication, namely written and verbal communication, and personal perception of members of the team of factors that might impede or enhance communication. Specific statements of intent such as this help at the next stage of the research which would be to design the research instruments that will be used to collect data as they define the parameters of the study (see Chapter 9).

Let us now consider some of the practical areas where this approach may be useful. One very commonly used approach to descriptive research in health care commonly falls under the management of quality of care. It is now very common in health care practice to ask people who use the service to comment on the service they have received. So in your day-to-day work you might ask your patients or clients to respond to questionnaires. The information or data collected from these surveys is collated, or gathered together, to give you an overall picture of the quality of service you provide. You might find when you read reports from these kind of surveys that patients express great satisfaction with some aspect of care and less satisfaction with other aspects of care. Overall you may feel quite pleased with the areas of satisfaction. Hence, when it comes to planning ways of service delivery you may focus on the results from the areas in which the patients are less satisfied and seek to improve those. At a simple level, this illustrates the utility value of descriptive research. It can give a useful snapshot of people's views of a situation at a given time.

You can of course extend this to other situations in health care. Imagine, for example, the situation where a member of a health care team feels that the skill mix in his or her area of practice was not right for the level of care required by the patient/client group and that to improve this it would be useful to present some facts to the manager of that unit. This practitioner might decide to undertake a small-scale study in which he or she asks staff about the types of task they do and the types of task they think they should be doing. In so doing he or she may find that the results differ from expectations; for example, that there is an overlap of activities undertaken by physiotherapists and nurses in some aspects of care, let us say rehabilitation. Alternatively, the practitioner may note that there is a difference between numbers of staff available with the skills required to do the tasks the practitioners feel should be done and those that are able to do them in practice. Asking people to comment on these issues can yield a lot of useful data: there is no need to manipulate the situation in any way to identify any deficit between what staff feel should be done and what they actually do. Yet, again, on the basis of the data from descriptive study, the data can be used by managers planning the service and looking to change practice.

It may be useful to explore this example in relation to another aspect of care. In undertaking this study the practitioner may realise that a lot of time is wasted undertaking routine tasks that have been part of the traditional practices. Prior to the research study looking at the use of skills nobody had thought to question why certain activities were undertaken or, if they had, they had not followed the question with any objective line of enquiry. For example, many practitioners now question the need for them to undertake tasks such as administrative tasks that could be more effectively carried out by a skilled administrator. If in the course of observations the researcher noted that a large amount of time was spent on paperwork which could be delegated to other personnel, he or she would be able to advise management of this and recommend adjustment in clerical support available to enable clinical practitioners to use their skills appropriately. This would perhaps be more cost effective in using the right level of skill for the job.

If practitioners are able to present a well-researched problem to the administrators they will stand a much stronger chance of improving the situation than if they rely simply on rhetoric and emotional arguments and assumed knowledge based on traditional practice rather than the facts of the situation observed (see Chapter 5).

Techniques of data collection in quantitative descriptive research

The techniques of data collection will be discussed in Chapter 9 but it should be noted here that researchers using descriptive approaches can draw on the range of techniques or data collection we have identified already, that is questionnaire, interviews and observations, and records. Out of these perhaps the most common approach is the questionnaire used as a *survey*. Surveys are such a popular method of collecting data to describe particular aspects of a phenomenon that they are commonly classed as research methods in their own right. Indeed there are very few people in the United Kingdom who would have got through life without being asked to participate in a survey, be that the national census, the market researcher who comes to your front door asking for your views on particular products, or the leaflets that drop through your letter box asking for your views on particular things. All of these constitute descriptive design because they are simply identifying your views in relation to a specific topic. Thus, for example, when we read the report of the national census we can find out how many people live in their own homes, how many homes are single occupancy and so on. Data presented from such surveys simply describe what is observed yet they have good utility value in identifying trends. For example, the national census helps in society by identifying trends that can be used with planning, such as housing needs for the future and so on.

Data analysis in quantitative descriptive designs

In the section above reference was made to using questionnaire surveys and observation tools to collect data in descriptive designs. Such data may be collected in a format that allows people to respond in a structured way to the questions asked and, in so doing, enables the researcher to analyse the data in numerical form. For example, if you have ever participated in a survey you will be familiar with the limited range of responses offered to questions – you might be constrained to a 'yes', 'no' or 'don't know' for example. We will return to the types of questions that may be used in tools used to collect data in descriptive research in Chapter 9. The important issue here is to note that the way in which data are analysed in a descriptive design reflects the purpose of the study, the aim being to describe the situation observed. As the data are quantitative they are analysed numerically using statistics, which are simply a way of summarising data. In this type of design *descriptive statistics*, which is simply a way of summarising our data in numerical form, is used (see Chapter 10).

Sample selection in descriptive design

The principles of sampling outlined in Chapter 6 apply to quantitative research design. Researchers using this approach endeavour to use a *random sample* approach to ensure that any views they gather are representative of the population they are studying. Where this is not possible, a sample of convenience may be used with the acknowledgement that it makes the finding less reliable if endeavouring to relate it to the population as whole.

In summary, descriptive research has a value in exploring situations and endeavouring to describe the 'here and now' in terms of people's attitudes, views or opinions relating to a given phenomenon or area of research interest. The value of taking a structured approach that lends itself to quantification is useful in that the views of large numbers of people can be gathered quickly and, depending on the design of the tools used for data collection, analysed relatively quickly.

Whilst descriptive research design is a widely used approach in research, however, there are times when researchers want more information from their data and it is the quest for more in-depth information that leads them from research which describes what is observed to research that facilitates the testing of any tentative theory that might have been formulated.

You will recall from Chapter 5 that there are several 'levels' of knowledge development from identifying concepts, to proposing relationships between them to testing whether these relationships really do exist. In descriptive research we are generally asking questions of an exploratory nature, questions that help to clarify concepts and perhaps, if comparing sets of data as in *comparative research*, beginning to identify some tentative relationships between the concepts.

Research designs that test proposed relationships

To enable us to test out developing ideas or developing theories we need to move to other ways of developing research, namely *correlational* and *experimental* research designs. To do this we develop a hypothesis, and this is something we need to consider before moving on to the other types of quantitative research design.

Hypothesis testing

A hypothesis, abbreviated to H_1, is a way of proposing a relationship between two or more variables, or factors, being studied. So for example we might propose the following hypothesis:

> There is a relationship between the level of patient satisfaction and the skill level of practitioners

In this hypothesis we have proposed a relationship between two variables, the first variable, patient satisfaction, and the second variable, the skill level of staff. The point to note in this hypothesis is that we have simply suggested that *there is a relationship* between the two variables. This is the kind of hypothesis we might use when developing a correlation research design – we will return to this below.

The kind of hypothesis we develop in experimental research design will be more specific and clearly identify at least two variables known as the *independent variable* and the *dependent* variable. The hypothesis predicts that the *independent* variable will *cause* an *effect* on the *dependent* variable. So for example a researcher might state:

> Exposure to cold weather will result in an increase in hypothermia in elderly people

In this instance the cold weather is the independent variable as this will affect the level of hypothermia, the dependent variable. Logically it could not be the other way around, for to do so would be to state that 'hypothermia will have an effect on cold weather' which sounds quite nonsensical. The point to remember is that the independent variable will cause an effect on the dependent variable as illustrated in the following hypotheses:

> Excess exposure to the sun will cause the skin to burn
>
> High grades in the exam are a result of good quality teaching
>
> Limb stretching exercises will increase speed in running

In these examples exposure to the sun is the independent variable as it will cause an effect on the skin (the skin will burn). In the second example the quality of teaching is the independent variable; it is proposed this will affect the exam grades. In the third example the limb stretching exercises are the independent variable for it is proposed these will have an effect on running speed, the dependent variable.

It would be useful for you to note that other terms used to refer to the hypothesis are the *experimental hypothesis* and the *alternative hypothesis*.

Null hypothesis

Another term you need to be familiar with is the null hypothesis, commonly abbreviated to H_0. The *null hypothesis* is a statement, a prediction of null effect, or no relationship between the variables. For a number of philosophical reasons the null hypothesis provides the basis for statistical testing. At an introductory level you do not need to understand these reasons but you do need to be able to formulate a null hypothesis if you are going to develop a study to test a hypothesis.

When using statistical tests to test a hypothesis the researcher is, in effect, seeking support for the null hypothesis. If the null hypothesis is accepted, then the hypothesis is rejected as false; if the null hypothesis is rejected, then the hypothesis is accepted as true. To illustrate this, refer to the examples which were written as hypotheses above and are now presented as null hypotheses:

> Excess exposure to the sun will have no effect on the skin
>
> The grades in the exam will not be influenced by the quality of teaching
>
> Limb stretching exercises will have no effect on speed in running

Note that in each of these the emphasis has varied from a positive statement proposing a relationship in the hypotheses above to one in which a negative relationship, or a statement of no effect, has been proposed in the null hypothesis. So, if we were to accept the null hypothesis that excess exposure to the sun will have no effect on the skin we would be rejecting the hypothesis above and so on. If you decide to undertake a study that will test a hypothesis you therefore need to be able to reword this to formulate the null hypothesis.

One-tailed and two-tailed hypotheses

In the examples above it has been suggested that the independent variable will have a specific effect on the dependent variable, that is, it will 'cause the skin to burn', result in high exam grades or 'increase the speed of running'. Sometimes when developing a research study it is not appropriate to be so specific about the kind of impact on the dependent variable. For example a researcher might think that teaching style may affect exam grades but may not be so confident that this will increase the grades. In this case he or she might state:

> The quality of the teaching will have an effect on the exam grades achieved

Whilst this hypothesis is stating that there will be an effect on the independent variable (the exam grades) it does not state the specific *direction* of that effect. The independent variable, teaching style, could cause an effect on the dependent variable in two directions, that is it could increase the grades achieved or it might decrease the exam grades achieved. This is known as a two-tailed hypothesis as the outcome could be in one of two directions. We could rephrase the other two examples to make them into two-tailed hypotheses as follows:

> Excess exposure to the sun will have an effect on the skin

> Limb stretching exercises will affect speed in running

In the first example it is suggested that excess exposure to the sun will have an effect on the skin but we are not stating what this is, whether the skin will burn or not. Likewise the notion of the exercises having an effect on running is less specific: it could be to increase the speed but it could also decrease speed.

So why do you need to know about one-tailed and two-tailed hypotheses? The reason is linked to the way in which you will develop and interpret your statistical tests. The outcome of a two-tailed test is less specific than a one-tailed test and this is reflected in the final analysis in statistical testing. We will return to this point in Chapter 10.

Correlational research designs

Correlational research designs serve to answer rather more detailed questions than that of descriptive research design. The researcher using this approach will not only want to identify the descriptive components of the situation observed but will also want to ask the question, 'What is the relationship between these factors or variables that I am observing?'. This point can be illustrated if we develop our examples above. Consider a situation in which a researcher asks the question 'Is there a relationship between patient satisfaction and the skill mix available in the health care team?'. The starting point therefore may be a hypothesis which proposes a relationship between variables as follows:

> There is a relationship between the level of patient satisfaction and the skill level of practitioners

To examine this the researcher may collect data from patients to determine their level of satisfaction. At the same time he or she could collect data from the practitioners to determine the level of skill available. Note that in this situation the researcher is simply collecting data – thus far the processes involved are the same as descriptive research design, there is no attempt to manipulate the situation that is being researched; both patients and staff are simply being asked to respond to questions relating to satisfaction (the patients) and skill mix available (for practitioners). In correlational design, however, the way in which the data are analysed is different.

Data collection and analysis in correlational design

The researcher using correlational approaches will perhaps start with descriptive statistics to summarise the responses from each group. Then he or she will move on to another level of analysis in which the findings from each group of responses are compared to see if they correlate with each other in any way. So, in our example, the researcher might look to see if patient satisfaction is associated with the level of skill in staff on the clinical area. In this case there are several possible outcomes:

1. A high level of patient satisfaction relates to a high level of skill available.
2. A low level of patient satisfaction relates to a low level of skill available.
3. A high level of patient satisfaction relates to a low level of skill available.
4. A low level of patient satisfaction relates to a high level of skill available.
5. There may be no relationship between the level of patient satisfaction and the skill mix.

So how do we know whether there is a relationship between the variables studied? At a very simple level you can do this by simply looking at the results of your analysis. Let us say you asked the patients to indicate their level of satisfaction by indicating on a five-point scale whether they were satisfied with the care they received. A score of 5 might indicate a high level of satisfaction and a score of 1 might indicate they were very dissatisfied as indicated below:

Please indicate the level of satisfaction you feel about your care by circling the response that indicates your feelings below where 5 = very satisfied and 1 = very dissatisfied:

     very satisfied   5   4   3   2   1   very dissatisfied

Given this example we can see that a high score indicates a high level of satisfaction. The maximum score that could be given to a singe respondent is 5 so the maximum possible total score for ten people would be 50 as $10 \times 5 = 50$.

At a descriptive level we can count the results from each person and give an overall score to indicate levels of patient satisfaction. Thus if we were to collate the results from ten patients and found the overall score was 45 we might conclude that most respondents (in this case the patient group) scored near or at 5 and so this represents a high level of satisfaction. Alternatively if we were to collate the results for ten patients and found the overall score was 10 you could conclude that this group were very dissatisfied as the minimum score per person would be 1 and $10 \times 1 = 10$.

The same process can be completed with their scores from the staff in relation to skill mix. We could ask staff to respond as follows:

On the scale below please indicate whether you feel the staffing levels today indicate a good skill mix for the care required for your patients where 5 = a high level of skill and 1 = a low level of skill

high level of skill   5   4   3   2   1   low level of skill

In this example if ten nurses scored a total of 45 we might assume that they felt there was a high level of skill. Likewise if ten nurses scored 1 to give a total of 10 we might assume that they thought there was a low level of skill available.

Now you can see how the scores might be worked out you can return to the potential outcomes from this small study. It was suggested above that there could be five outcomes to this study and that you could determine if there was a relationship in the first instance by simply looking at your responses. If the responses from ten patients totalled 45 and the response about the level of skill from ten nurses totalled 45 you might conclude there was a relationship between patient satisfaction and the level of skill mix. As both sets of data have a high score this would be described as a *positive correlation* as a high score on one is associated with a high score on the other set of data. If, in contrast, the patients' score was 10 and the nurses' score was 45 you might conclude there was a relationship but in this case it would be a *negative correlation* because there is a low score on the patients' response and a high score to the nurses' response.

In our example we have been discussing a very small sample of respondents, ten nurses and ten patients. Given such numbers it is relatively easy to look at the overall score and identify patterns in the data. However, if data are more detailed and the numbers of respondents greater, it is not so easy to observe relationships 'at a glance'. Consider, for example, what might happen if you asked 100 patients and 100 nurses to respond to your questions. The results from a study with such large numbers would be more complex to analyse. So, you might want to use a computer to help you to analyse your data.

Also, you want to know whether any relationships you are observing in the data are important. In the samples referred to above it was suggested that there was an apparent relationship in the data, but to know whether this was the case you would need to undertake some statistical tests which will tell you whether the results you are looking at are due to 'chance' or whether there is a real relationship between the two sets of data, that is whether they are *significant* results. To know whether results are significant you need to undertake some statistical tests. The tests you use in correlational research design are simply called *correlational statistical tests*. We will return to these in Chapter 10.

In summary, correlational research design can be used to help us to identify whether there is a relationship between variables observed in research. The important point to remember in correlational design is that the results can only indicate whether or not there is a relationship. If there is a relationship it can only be reported as such – you cannot claim that a relationship observed in a correlational study is an indication of cause and effect. The reason for this is that in correlational design the researcher has not exerted any control or manipulation over the variables studied. So in the example above we could note a high score on patient satisfaction and a high score on skill mix available and we could conclude that there was a relationship. We could not however state that the high level of patient satisfaction was *caused* by the high level of skill available. This might have been due to a host of other things that we had not considered in the research. For example, if we had asked the patients if they owned a television set, a high number may say 'yes'. We could then perhaps have identified a correlation between satisfaction and owning a television set! The important point here is that any research design you choose to do will have very specific guidelines to enable you to avoid such obvious pitfalls. It is important that you follow such guidelines with care to ensure that any interpretation in correlation design is made with caution.

Experimental research designs

The purpose of experimental research design is to identify 'causal relationships', that is whether the independent variable has an effect on the dependent variable. Consequently experimental research approaches are designed in such a way that the researcher is able to test the hypothesis by observing the *effect* of the *independent variable* on the *dependent variable*.

A true experimental design has three characteristics which make this approach distinct from other approaches discussed earlier:

1. The selection of the sample group is always *random*.
2. The researcher is active in *manipulating* some aspect of the research.
3. The researcher sets the parameters to the study by exerting *control*.

Randomisation

Random sampling procedures mean that every member of a given population has an equal chance of participating in the research (see Chapter 6). The purpose of randomisation is to ensure that, as far as possible, the effects on the dependent variable can be attributed to the independent variable.

In any group of people being studied the researcher will know there are some aspects that might make a difference to the outcome of the research. These are referred to as *extraneous variables* and can thus be defined as any variable other than the independent variable which may influence the effect on the dependent variable to be measured. Random sampling procedures imply that this can be done by excluding those variables that might impact on the outcome of the research.

Whilst this depends on the nature of the research project there are some things that might be seen as potential *extraneous variables* in a population that may influence the research design. For example, people of different ages will respond differently to different things, sex and ethnicity might make a difference in the way in which we respond to the world around us. In addition to those things the researcher can identify as causing a potential problem in research there are other things that might impact on the results of a study, sometimes unknown factors can influence the outcome – so the argument is that selecting a random sample will help avoid the impact of other variables on the study.

For example, if the doctor undertaking a research study to determine the effectiveness of a new headache tablet wanted to identify a group of people for study, this sample would need to be drawn from the defined population, in the first instance in a random way. In this case the population would be those people suffering from headache. This may be by allocating a number to each potential respondent or simply by picking names out of a hat.

Manipulation

This describes the situation where the researcher is *active* in the research process and does something to at least some of the people being studied. For example, a physiotherapist testing a new exercise regime will introduce that regime to the client group, a doctor carrying out a trial of new drugs will prescribe the new drugs to the people participating in the experimental study, a nurse exploring new models of care will expose some of his or her patients to the new model. In this context reference is sometimes made to the *condition* which is the situation under which participants are being studied.

Control

In experimental design researchers introduce some control over the study by eliminating the influences of those variables other than those being manipulated by the researcher on the dependent variable. So for example a physiotherapist testing a new exerciser regime would need to know that this was the only programme his or her client was following. The doctor testing a new drug for headaches would, in a true experiment, endeavour to ensure that the person testing the new drug was not taking any other painkillers that would mask the effect of the new drug. Other potential variables that might influence the outcome of the research need to be considered and excluded. For example, in the drug trial other factors that might impact on a person's perception of pain might be the type of pain he or she has (chronic or acute), age and ethnicity (as it is known that pain thresholds vary across ethnic groups). Anticipating such variables means that the risk of error in the research results can be reduced, although, as noted above, random errors, or errors due to chance, will be of concern and considered when the statistical test are developed.

Types of experimental design

The basic principles of experimental research can therefore be seen as being able to ensure the sample is selected on a basis of randomisation and that the researcher can manipulate the independent variable in a controlled situation. There are, however, other things that the experimental researcher needs to consider when planning how to test a hypothesis; that is, to measure if the independent variable causes an effect on the dependent variable.

The first point to make here is that the process of randomisation needs to consider ways in which *bias* can be excluded from the findings from a group. There are several ways of doing this, each offering a more 'refined' approach.

To start with the researcher will need to clarify exactly what is to be measured and how the measuring is going to be carried out. What to measure is determined by the hypothesis. Refer to the example in which we stated the hypothesis that

High grades in the exam are a result of good quality teaching.

In this example the concepts that will be measured will be 'high grades' and 'good quality teaching' and the researcher would need to define exactly what he or she understood by using these terms. Failure to be specific about this could lead to confusion later in the study.

The most simple way of testing this hypothesis will be to complete a *simple pre-test, post-test design*. Remember that the teaching is the independent variable and the grades in the exam are the dependent variable. In such a study the researcher would measure the student grades before the 'high quality teaching' (the pre-test on the dependent variable) and after the teaching experience (the post-test of the dependent variable). If the grades increased markedly between the pre- and post-test the researcher might suggest this was due to the quality of the teaching (the independent variable).

However, you might feel a little uneasy about this and have some questions you would like to ask. First you would want to be sure that the student exposed to the high quality teaching had been randomly selected to ensure an appropriate mix of intelligence. A teacher going into a group of students who have high IQs might not be surprised if the grades were high following the teaching experience regardless of the 'quality' of the teaching. Secondly you might want to know what was meant by 'high quality teaching'. This is a more elusive concept than high or low exam grades and, as indicated earlier, the definition needs to be clearly spelt out.

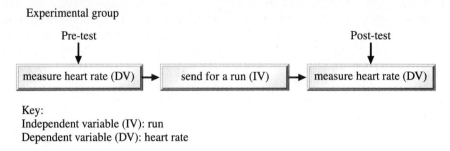

Figure 8.3 Example of pre-test, post-test design.

So, to recap, the basic model of experimental design is one of randomisation, manipulation and control. Within this, if measures of the effect of the independent variable on the dependent variable are to be clear then clear definition of what constitutes these variables is required. Look, for example, at Figure 8.3 in which we have illustrated the hypothesis 'running will increase the heart rate'. This is more straightforward than the above as our independent variable here is running and our dependent variable, the heart rate. In this example the experimental group will be exposed to the treatment or condition of the independent variable and expected to 'run'. The researcher would need to be sure that they could describe exactly what they meant by a 'run' – how might this differ from fast walking for example. The dependent variable, the heart rate, is relatively straightforward to describe and determine ways of measuring. This form of study is known as a *within-subject design*

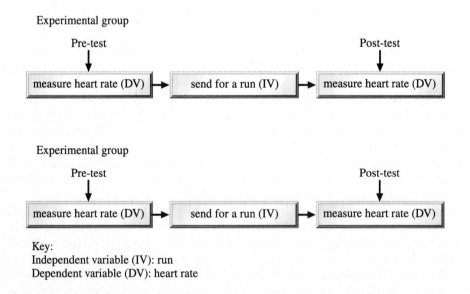

Figure 8.4 Example of pre-, post-test study using control group.

| Experimental group | R | O_1 | | X | O_2 |
| Control group | R | O_1 | | | O_2 |

Key: R   =   randomisation
       O   =   observation (of dependent variable)
       X   =   treatment or intervention (independent variable)
       O_1 =   pre-test
       O_2 =   post-test

Figure 8.5 Experimental model.

because the same group is being used in both the pre- and post-test.

This brings us back to randomisation of subjects. If we were proposing that running will increase heart rate we would want to know if this can be generalised to the population as a whole. So, the experimental group is randomly selected and the situation controlled and manipulated. However, we need to be sure that any change in heart rate is not due to other variables that we have not considered, so-called *extraneous variables*. For example, the level of fitness of the person running might influence the heart rate measured. This refers to any variable other than the independent variable which may influence the effect on the dependent variable to be measured. To do this the researcher would introduce a *control group* which is a second group that will not be exposed to the independent variable but will be subject to the same measures of the dependent variable as the experimental group (see Figure 8.4). If on completion of a study a difference is observed this may be accounted for by the impact of the independent variable on the dependent variable in the experimental group. However, as you will see in Chapter 10, this conclusion would be confirmed or refuted by statistical tests.

You need to remember that in addition to the manipulation of the independent variable and use of a control group there is still a need to ensure that the sample is randomly selected. The *experimental model* is therefore commonly presented as indicated in Figure 8.5.

Once different groups are introduced into a research study the researcher can be more specific about the sample or subjects involved. So the term *different subject design* is used to indicate an approach in which each group takes part in the study by participating in one condition or treatment only, as illustrated in Figure 8.5. This can be developed further and the different subjects can be 'matched' as far as possible on the variables that might influence the study. For example, if doing a study to determine the impact of a new educational programme on the experimental group you might wish to match your subject group (a *matched subject design*) in terms of factors that could bias the results. In this case it might be age, educational experience or attainment.

This experimental model can be extended to include a wider range of observations if necessary and so in health care research you may read of researchers undertaking studies in which there may be more than one experimental group and thus more than one treatment regime. Reports of such studies may refer to different 'arms' of

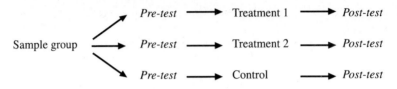

Figure 8.6 Example of experimental design with more than one treatment arm.

the research to indicate different exposures as indicated in Figure 8.6. If the studies in each treatment group are going on at the same time, they may be referred to as 'parallel studies'. Researchers commonly use such terms in research reports to indicate the research design used; so if you were to read that a research study was 'a randomly controlled, experimental, parallel research study using two treatment arms' you should be able to work out exactly what happened to each group. Such descriptions are not uncommon in drug trials.

Crossover designs

One of the risks of experimental design is that respondents may change their behaviour simply because they are the focus of interest. For example, consider if a researcher was testing a new drug for headache. If this was a new drug it is possible that the person might assume it was a better treatment than anything tried before and so the impact of their belief might relieve the headache. This is known as the *placebo effect*. For this reason *crossover designs* are adopted in some experimental studies to try to avoid the effect of the independent variable being influenced by factors other than the independent variable. In crossover designs efforts are made to check the impact by observing the outcome of the independent variable in two or more groups of subjects as illustrated in Figure 8.7. The same principles of undertaking pre- and post-tests, would apply and measures would be completed at each stage of the study.

In health care you will commonly see this in experimental studies examining the effectiveness of new drugs – so called drug trials. If a doctor or pharmacist was developing a study to examine the impact of a new headache drug he or she could adopt a simple experimental design as indicated in Figure 8.5. However, it is possible that any positive results generated by such a study may be due to the time at which the drug was administered – perhaps immediately finishing another painkilling regime of drugs. By introducing a crossover design the subjects will be told when they enter the study that they will be exposed to the independent variable (the trial drug) or a placebo (a substitute that has similar properties to the independent variable). Consequently when measures are made of the dependent variable it might be anticipated that, if the independent variable is the cause of any changes, the results from the group taking the trial drug would differ from the results of the placebo group. However, two issues arise out of this. The first one is that the order in which the experimental treatment is administered may influence the outcome. This is known

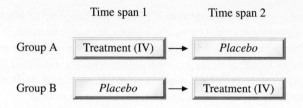

Figure 8.7 Illustration of a crossover design.

as the *order effect* which is defined as a measurable change in participants in an experimental study that may result from their experiencing one treatment condition before another. So this is another issue that should be considered in the context of the placebo effect.

Secondly, the subject may not know which drugs they are receiving (i.e. they are *blind* to treatment). It is possible that if the researcher is aware of the treatment at the time (that is the active drug or the placebo) this may affect the way he or she approaches the person. A little innuendo about a particular treatment being especially beneficial could lead a subject (participating in a research trial) to think that this phase was the treatment phase – again this could potentially affect the outcome. So, to avoid this, the concept of '*a double blind trial*' is commonly adopted in health care research, particularly in drug trials. In this instance neither the person receiving the treatment nor the person giving the treatment will know which treatment is being administered.

It is important to note that when double blind trials are being developed there are particular ethical concerns that need to be addressed. This lies primarily in the nature of the study and the problem area on which the study is focusing. Let us say the study was focusing on a new drug to control blood pressure. The question is, what happens if the person participating in the trial starts to develop problems with blood pressure and neither the doctor leading the trial nor the patient knows whether they are receiving anti-hypertensive drugs or a placebo? The answer to this is that there must be some way of identifying the drugs involved in the trial at any time in the study and such a mechanism is usually incorporated in the project design. The information can usually be obtained through a third person such as a pharmacist distributing the drugs but not in direct contact with the research subject.

Strengths and weaknesses of experimental design

Experimental design is the most powerful method of testing hypotheses. Some aspects of research only lend themselves to this approach, for example, in health care, any research impacting on physiological work. However, there are also a number of limitations. Firstly, there are a high number of variables not amenable to manipulation.

For example, whilst we can manipulate physiological aspects of humans it is not so easy to manipulate psychological aspects. Linked with this perhaps is the perspective that it may be possible to manipulate variables but not ethically acceptable to do so. Consider, for example, if a medical researcher who thought that certain chemical substances caused cancer. He or she would not be allowed to administer the substances to test the hypothesis as this would not be ethically acceptable.

Other considerations include the fact that in decontextualising a situation for the purposes of research it may not be 'typical' of how people would be treated normally. Consider, for example, the health promotion officer who wanted to complete a study into a health education programme. A pre-test would be done to determine the knowledge level for the sample group and then this would be followed up with a health promotion programme designed to inform the subjects about a certain aspect of health, say, keeping fit. A post-test would determine if the programme had been successful and on the basis of this the researcher might make recommendations for the future. But what we have to remember is that in the research situation the independent variable (the health promotion package) is being carefully controlled and manipulated by the researcher. In the real world there may not be sufficient health promotion officers to give such a detailed programme to the population at large – they might have to rely more heavily on written information and so on. Another consideration is the potential impact of the so-called *Hawthorne effect* – that is, the risk that people might change their behaviour simply on the basis of being observed.

Finally, it must be noted that in many health care situations it is not always feasible for researchers to complete experimental research studies. For nurses and health care workers in particular this is an important point, for experience has shown that trying to establish an experimental study in clinical areas sometimes requires an integration between so many members of a health care team that it becomes impossible.

Quasi-experimental research

Because of the difficulty in meeting the requirements of experimental design, a researcher in health care may need to resort to quasi-experimental research design which, as the title implies, is the kind of study that reflects an experimental design but not completely so. In quasi-experimental design the researcher will manipulate the independent variable but lack one or both other characteristics of experimental design, that is control or randomisation. Consequently quasi-experimental design is weaker than experiment in noting cause and effect.

Quasi-experimental research has some advantages including practicality and feasibility and although acknowledged as being weaker than experimental design, the findings can to some extent be generalised to a wider population. The major weakness in quasi-experimental design lies in the fact that the observed effect on the dependent variable may be due to a rival 'hypothesis' because of the limitations introduced by a lack of random sampling procedures. Consequently it is hard to prove cause and effect.

Techniques of data collection in experimental design

Instruments used for data collection in experimental research design need very careful development to ensure that measures of the variables are both *valid* (that is measuring what they are supposed to measure) and *reliable* (consistent in their measurement). Techniques of data collection may include questionnaires (self-administered or face-to-face interview) or observation or other forms of data relevant to the particular study, for example, checklists to indicate physiological measures. Whatever techniques are used, the features of such studies are that they need to be developed in such a way that data can be quantified to enable the statistical testing required to compare the pre-test data with post-test data.

So in research studies involving 'pre-test and post-test' the researcher gathers base line data at the beginning of the study by measuring the dependent variable, introduces the independent variable to the sample and then proceeds to measure the dependent variable again. Any measurable changes to the dependent variable *may* then be credited to the influence of the independent variable.

Data analysis in experimental design

The researcher will test the hypothesis by using appropriate statistical tests. As you will see in Chapter 10 different statistical tests will be used for different types of research design discussed above. For example, descriptive statistics are used for descriptive research design and inferential statistics are used in experimental design. Inferential statistics enable the researcher to determine if any differences in the data are due to the intervention of the independent variable or to chance.

In summary experimental research seeks to identify relationships between events. Unlike the situation in the school laboratory outlined in Chapter 1, in which chemical substances can be manipulated to identify a cause and effect relationship, in health care research the subject matter is more commonly people and situations related to their health. This may be one of the reasons why the experimental approach has not been as widely adopted as descriptive research. In manipulating situations in relation to people controlling variables can be difficult and ethical dilemmas can arise.

ACTIVITY _____

- Consider an area of your work in which a quantitative study could be carried out.
- State what type of quantitative study you would use for your example (descriptive, correlational, experimental).
- How would you collect the data for your study?
- What do you think might be the strengths and limitations of the approach you have chosen?

- Try writing two or three hypotheses related to your area of work.
- Now change these hypotheses to null hypotheses.

Summary

This chapter has explored a range of research designs that quantify data in some form. This includes descriptive research design, correlational research design and experimental research designs.

Further reading

Brockopp, D.Y. and Hastings-Tolsma, M.T. (1995) *Fundamentals of Nursing Research*, 2nd edn, Jones & Bartlett, Boston.

Clark, E. (1991) *Research Awareness Module 8 The Survey Perspective,* Distance Learning Centre, South Bank Polytechnic (South Bank University), London.

Clark, E. (1991) *Research Awareness Module 9 The Experimental Perspective*, Distance Learning Centre, South Bank Polytechnic (South Bank University), London.

Cormack, D.F.S. (1991) *The Research Process in Nursing*, 2nd edn, Blackwell Scientific, Oxford.

Fowler, F.J. (1993) *Survey Research Methods*, 2nd edn, Sage, London.

Hicks, C. (1990) *Research and Statistics: A Practical Introduction for Nurses.* Prentice Hall, Hemel Hempstead.

Hinton, P.R. (1995) *Statistics Explained: A Guide for Social Science Students*, Routledge, London.

Keeble, S. (1995) *Experimental Research 1 and 2*, Open Learning Foundation, Churchill Livingstone, Edinburgh.

Reid, N. (1993) *Health Care Research by Degrees*, Blackwell Scientific, Oxford.

See also: 'Experimental Research', *Nurse Researcher*, vol. 1, no. 4, June (1994).

9   Techniques used in data collection

This chapter gives an outline of some of the techniques used by researchers to gather data. The chapter will cover the commonest means of data collection in health care research which fall into the following categories:

1. Questionnaires.
2. Interviews.
3. Observation.
4. Other techniques of data collection.

Collecting data in qualitative and quantitative research

The techniques of data collection described in this chapter can be used in both qualitative and quantitative research. However, as you will see below, the qualitative researcher will be likely to collect data in an apparently less structured way than the quantitative researcher. The issues of 'structure' is one commonly used in research to indicate the format of data collection. A 'high level of structure' in data collection implies that the research instrument is designed in such a way that the range of data collected is prescribed at the outset. In contrast a 'low level of structure' suggests that the range of data collected cannot be predicted at the outset: it is dependent on the person or situation being studied. Generally speaking the level of 'structure' in a research tool is linked to the orientation of the research, that is whether it is quantitative or qualitative. Tools used in quantitative studies tend to be highly structured as they seek to gather very specific data that can be quantified in some way. The researcher will know at the outset the range of responses that will be gathered from respondents. In contrast tools used in qualitative studies have less structure as they are used to get the individual perspective of the people participating in the research. Here, the emphasis is on obtaining the views of the participants and so the researcher is less able to predict what the respondents will say in response to questions asked. It is, of course, possible to ask questions in qualitative research in an ordered or a structured sequence. Consequently, the degree of structure in a research tool used will depend also on the extent to which the questions asked or the observations undertaken are 'open or closed'. *Open questions* allow respondents in research to respond in their own words, to tell the researcher exactly what they see or feel about the things they are asked to comment on (low structure). In contrast, *closed questions* ask for a very specific response to a question and those responding to such questions are faced with a limited range of responses (high structure).

The same principles can be applied to observations in research. An open observation technique would involve the researcher in recording what is seen in such a way that impressions are recorded as they arise. In contrast a highly structured or 'closed' observation study would enable the researcher to make very specific measurable observations, such as, for example, measuring time taken to perform a specific task, of very specific actions taken to complete a task. In this case the researcher knows exactly what he or she is going to record at the outset.

In addition to the use of 'open and closed' approaches, researchers sometimes refer to the use of a 'semi-structured' approach to data collection. This may be indicative of a mixture of open and closed questions within a research tool or indicate the use of open questions in a structured sequence.

Types of data

Open approaches to data collection will generate data in words that will be subject to qualitative approaches of data analysis. We discuss this further in the next chapter. The more structured data generated through closed questioning techniques can be further divided into categories to indicate the type of data collected:

1. Nominal.
2. Ordinal.
3. Interval/ratio.

Nominal data are those that can be grouped into named categories. An example of this would be sex (male, female) but any other category that can be named could be included. For example whether people are smokers or non-smokers, play sports or do not play sports and so on.

Ordinal data are also data that can be allocated to named categories but in this instance data may be 'ordered'. An example of this could be whether people are non-smokers, light smokers, medium smokers or heavy smokers. These data can be ordered to indicate the level of smoking.

Interval/ratio data are data that can be measured on a scale where the distance between each point is identical. So for example you might want to note how many cigarettes respondents smoke and so you might develop a scale that identifies whether they smoke ten a day, twenty a day, thirty a day and so on. The important distinction here is that the difference between each measure is very precise, as in our example above where each measure can be described in units of ten.

It should be noted that interval and ratio measures are different in that ratio measures have an absolute zero measure. However, as there are 'equal measures between points on the scale' in both measures, they are referred to together for the purpose of analysis in a number of statistical tests.

The reason you need to consider these types of data at the outset of designing any research instruments is that the way in which you develop your data analysis will be clearly influenced by the type of data you have collected. There are specific statistical tests used for different types of data and one of the important points in research design is that you consider each stage of the research whilst planning your study. So, as you are developing the research instruments you wish to use, you need also to be considering how you will analyse the data. This point applies equally to both quantitative and qualitative data.

We will now consider these issues in the context of each approach to data collection, questionnaires, interviews and observations.

Using questionnaires in research

Questionnaires can be used to collect data in the range of research designs discussed in previous chapters. The overall research design will determine the type of information you want to collect, qualitative or quantitative, and what you will do with the data gathered by questionnaires. For example, in a descriptive study, data will be used to describe the situation observed, whilst in a correlational study data will be used to look for relationships between variables. In experimental research data would be collected at both pre- and post-test to determine the impact of the independent variable on the dependent variable.

The use of questionnaires allows the researcher to gather facts or opinions related to a given topic. In gathering opinions questionnaires are seen as a good medium for measuring attitudes, motivation or values of respondents. In addition they are frequently used to predict events. For example, one form of prediction that we are all familiar with is that of predicting the outcome of general elections. The avid news watcher at general election time will not only be used to hearing what the trends are in terms of public attitudes towards particular political parties but will have noted that the reporting of these has become rather more sophisticated as public awareness of research methods used has increased. Now news reports carry not only the results of various attitude surveys but proceed to describe the sample size and location of the study. This allows those alert to research techniques to consider the appropriateness of sampling techniques and any potential for bias.

In health care research the use of questionnaires to undertake a study has been very popular. The advantages of undertaking this approach do, to some extent, explain why this method is favoured. These are outlined in more detail below. At this stage, however, it is worth making a note of caution. Newcomers to research often think that it is easy to undertake a 'quick' research study by producing a questionnaire and circulating this to their sample group. What they realise very quickly is that, however good the research idea, it is actually very difficult to produce a good questionnaire. In research terms a questionnaire is not simply a set of questions randomly put together, rather it is an *instrument* or *tool* designed to explore specific research questions.

Designing a questionnaire

Some of the key points that should be considered when designing a questionnaire are outlined below. This is not intended to be a definitive guide, but it is included simply to increase awareness of the kind of issues that must be considered when using questionnaires in a research study. For further guidance on this you are referred to the further reading at the end of the chapter.

The first, and perhaps most important point, in questionnaire design is to be very clear of the purpose of the research study, what questions you are asking and what variable you want to measure. This will give you the focus required for developing questions. For example, if you have a set of clearly stated aims and objectives as in a descriptive quantitative research design, this will give a framework by which to develop several questions around each objective. If you have stated one or more hypotheses in a correlational or experimental design you will need to identify all the variables that derive from this hypothesis to consider how these should be included in the questionnaire.

The following points relate to some general considerations when developing questionnaires.

Presentation

It is very important that the initial presentation of a questionnaire is such that the respondent will not be immediately put off completing the questionnaire. A good guide in this would be to consider the difference between picking up a large print, easy-to-read book and one which is in tiny print and has very cramped pages. The former would be more appealing to the majority of people looking for a 'light read' whilst the latter would perhaps appeal only if the particular subject matter under review was of great interest to the reader. The questionnaire design should attract the interests of the majority of the group of respondents it is designed for.

The *layout* of the questionnaire is important. It is important to make the questionnaire presentable, easy to read and understand and easy to respond to. A well-spaced style of presentation is important both for the respondent and for the researcher when he or she does the analysis.

The amount of information required on the front sheet of the questionnaire should be considered. At the top of the page the researcher should indicate how he or she wants the respondents to complete the questionnaire, giving clear and unambiguous *instructions.*

It is a common practice, although not a rigid rule, to include any necessary *biographical detail* at the beginning of a questionnaire, although some texts advise this is left to the end of the questionnaire. Questions such as age, sex and place of work are usually addressed in the biographical section. Researchers must consider very carefully what information is included in this section and they should take care to ensure that only essential data are requested from respondents. Failure to do this may contribute towards '*non-compliance*' as respondents can be very easily put off completing questionnaires if they think questions are not related to the topic under review (see below). For example respondents may start filling out a questionnaire about their attitudes to work but, if faced with a question pertaining to a very personal aspect of their own life not apparently related to other aspects of the questionnaire, they may question the purpose of the study and stop their response because of this. They may suspect some ulterior motive behind seemingly irrelevant questions and, perhaps, question the integrity of the research.

The biographical section gives you an opportunity to consider the type of data you are collecting and the best way of doing so. For example you might want to know sex, occupation (nominal categories) or age range (interval/ratio categories). This latter category is important in helping you consider the fact that each response should be *mutually exclusive*, that is there should be no overlap between responses. For example, when asking respondents to indicate their age, newcomers to research may put the following categories:

> 20–30 years ☐   30–40 years ☐   40–50 years ☐

The problem with these categories is that the respondent who is 30- or 40-years-old would not know which box to tick; some 30-year-olds might choose the first and others would choose the second and so on. Consequently the data would not be very reliable if you wanted to use these categories to do some comparative or correlation analysis. The categories should look like those below, where you will note they have been made 'mutually exclusive' by containing more specific age ranges in each group:

> 20–30 years ☐   31–40 years ☐   41–50 years ☐

You will note that in each of the categories above small boxes have been positioned alongside the category to enable the respondent to tick their response. This is not essential as you will have come across questionnaires where you have been asked to 'circle' the correct response or 'delete those that are not relevant'. However, generally speaking, the tick box response demands less effort on the part of the respondent and certainly makes it easier for the researcher to note the specific response when it comes to analysing the data.

Explaining the purpose of the questionnaire to respondents

Respondents should be advised about the purpose of the study. If questionnaires are to be administered face to face it is easy for the researcher to give this information verbally. Failing that, some form of written explanation must be given. This can be done on the top of the questionnaire. Alternatively a short letter can be written to research subjects, explaining the purpose of the study, requesting co-operation and giving any relevant instructions relating to completion and the return of the questionnaire. A guarantee of anonymity is important to ensure that respondents know that confidentiality will be maintained. It is also courteous to thank respondents for participating in the study indicating, if possible, how, when and where the results of the study will be available to them.

Writing questions for use in a questionnaire

When developing questionnaires the way in which questions are phrased is very important. Questions should be clearly written and unambiguous and should relate to the stated aims of the research. There should not be anything within the structure of the question that will lead to a biased response. The researcher should avoid confusing the respondents by including questions that include negative statements, or worse, double negatives. For example if the respondent was asked to answer 'yes' or 'no' to the following question they may be rather confused:

> *Do you think it is not a good idea not to increase the length of hospital stay?*

This is not a good question because it is not clear to the respondent exactly what response is required. A better way of phrasing this would be:

> *Do you think it is a good idea to increase the patient's length of stay in hospital?*

You will find if you do develop a questionnaire that it is useful to ask someone else to review your questions for you. It is not uncommon for researchers to introduce ambiguities or bias into questions in the process of development.

Types of question

Writing questions for use in a questionnaire research is an important issue and not as easy as it first appears. Reference has already been made to the degree of structure in research and this is very evident in the kind of questions you might use. Low-structured questions are generally referred to as open questions and these are the type that will be used in questions that have a qualitative orientation. *Open questions* require the respondents to develop an individual response and so the potential range of information gathered using this approach can be quite large. Each statement made by an individual respondent will require in-depth analysis and will be subject to the methods described for content analysis in the next chapter. Open questions are developed in a way that invites 'open' response although the degree to which this is done can vary. For example an open question can ask a respondent to

> *'Explain what you feel about…'*

Alternatively an open question could ask respondents to

> *'List the three most important features of your job'*

The first of these questions is clearly qualitative in orientation although the latter will probably generate some responses that can be categorised in a more structured way. Here again consideration of how the information will be analysed is important when the questionnaire is being designed.

Questions that require a fixed response can be described as *closed questions*. The respondent only has a limited choice in the range of answers available. For example, a survey of the general public may be seeking to identify how many people are television owners. The question

'*Do you own a television set?*'

will demand a 'yes' or 'no' response. People either own a television set or they do not. However, this indicates the need to be cautious, for owning a television set is not an indication of whether or not people watch television and so further questioning would be required, if this was what you were trying to ascertain. It is quite easy to miss the obvious point such as this when immersed in your own questionnaire design. This again brings us back to the point of having clearly described the purpose to the study as, once a first draft of the questionnaire is completed it can be checked against your stated aims and variables to determine if they have all been covered in the questions asked.

Closed questions can also be used to enable respondents to express values, beliefs or feelings, but the way in which this is done is highly structured and employs a range of questioning styles as indicated below.

A variation of the closed question approach is the *forced choice*. The respondent is expected to make one of a number of choices from predetermined categories. This method could be used to determine if the respondent watches television once a day, once a month, once a year or never. Note that the type of data collected here is interval/ratio. This method does have some uses but can also be seen to be too limiting for some studies. In being forced to make a choice from one of the categories the respondent who watches television on a more erratic basis may be frustrated in trying to determine which of these responses fits his or her pattern of television watching.

A common example of a forced choice approach to determine attitudes is the Likert scale. These are scales developed from a variety of attitude statements pertaining to the area of study. Respondents are commonly asked to respond to a five-point scale which indicate the extent to which they agree with the statement as follows:

Strongly agree (SA)
Agree (A)
Uncertain (U)
Disagree (D)
Strongly disagree (SD)

The abbreviations in the brackets are commonly used in the actual questionnaire to help ensure a neat presentation – however, note that if they are used, the full meaning must be spelt out for respondents. As the Likert scale has some degree of order in terms of strength of response but does not have an exact measurement between categories this type of data is classed as ordinal.

Although Likert scales are widely used in health care research they demand a lot of development to ensure that they are a reliable measure of the phenomenon being studied, and so any reader wishing to develop this approach is recommended to the further reading at the end of the chapter.

Ranking scales are another example of recording responses in questionnaires. The respondent may be asked to indicate his or her strength of feeling on a given subject by ranking perceived priorities from most important to least important. These can be quite a useful means of indicating strength of feeling on a given topic, and in health care may make a useful contribution towards prioritising services, for example as illustrated below:

Please rank the following issues relating to your experiences in hospital where 1 = most important and 5 = least important:

☐   Good food
☐   Good communication with all staff
☐   Efficient treatment
☐   Open access for visitors
☐   Nice surroundings

It should be noted that whilst ranking scales are quite useful they are more complex to analyse in that the data may fall into nominal categories yet the ranking offers a degree of order that has not been predetermined by the researcher. So these need to be used with caution.

One other way of gathering data used in health care research that demands little effort from the respondent is the *visual analogue* scale which uses the impact of vision for data collection yet has the properties of an ordinal scale of measure in that data can be collated from least to most. This type of scale can be used to measure the 'level' related to the area of study, this might be satisfaction, happiness or pain, as illustrated below:

Please indicate by a mark on the scale below the amount of discomfort you have at present:

No   A lot of
discomfort   discomfort

───

This approach can be useful for studies with children or for those who do not read English well as the words can be replaced with visual images as indicated below:

To analyse the data generated in a visual analogue scale the researcher can develop an ordinal scale by marking out the scale at prescribed intervals. Commonly a 10 cm scale is used and, the 'score' taken from the point at which the respondent marks the scale.

All of these approaches outlined above represent methods which would facilitate quantitative research. The researcher will be able to measure in numerical terms how the respondents reacted to a given question.

Using mixed approaches to questionnaire design

Both quantitative and qualitative components can be used in questionnaires if open and closed questions are used in the same instrument. The mix of quantitative and qualitative methods may be quite useful in allowing some components of the data to be measured numerically then elaborating on these through open questions. In the final analysis the researcher will have quantitative information on which to base part of the report and this information can then be elaborated on by qualitative information available (see triangulation, Chapter 5).

Analysing questionnaire data

It is worth noting that, in principle, the easier it is for a respondent to complete a questionnaire then the easier it should be for the researcher to analyse the results. For example if, in a descriptive study, a questionnaire has a number of closed questions requiring simply a 'yes' or 'no' answer then all the researcher has to do is to count up the number of people who answered 'yes', the number who said 'no' and present the results. Equally, if the option is given for the respondents to reply to a number of statements which seek to identify attitudes by asking them to agree or disagree with the statements made, there is again a limited number of responses for the researcher to work with and the results are easily collated.

The important point here, however, is not the complexity of the analysis but consideration of the data which will be analysed at the outset. Newcomers to research quite frequently fall into the trap of setting a number of questions and not considering what they will do with the responses once they have been acquired. You should seek advice from a supervisor in the early stages of a research project to help you avoid this pitfall.

There are a number of ways questionnaires can be used, including self-completion and interviews. Each approach has advantages and disadvantages which will be discussed further below.

Self-administered questionnaires

A very popular way of using questionnaires is to ask the respondents to complete these themselves. Whilst there are a number of advantages of this approach there are also disadvantages of using this technique as you will see below.

Advantages of self-administered questionnaires

The use of self-administered questionnaires allows the researcher to get to a lot of people very quickly. It takes but a matter of minutes to circulate a handful of questionnaires to a sample of respondents to complete themselves. In contrast, if the researchers were to complete these themselves by asking the respondents the same questions using interview techniques it may take many hours, or even days, to acquire the same range of information from the same number of respondents. From this perspective it is easy to see why individual researchers may favour this method as it is feasible, in terms of time and effort, that one person could undertake quite a large-scale survey using questionnaires.

Another advantage is that the postal services can be used to reach a larger sample. Thus, for example, the health care researcher undertaking a study of clinical staff could circulate questionnaires to a random sample of 100 members of staff in several hospital or community units quite easily. Alternatively, if undertaking a study of patient satisfaction, it would be relatively easy to circulate 100 questionnaires to patients who have been discharged from hospital. It would be unrealistic for similar sample sizes to be obtained by the individual researcher using interview techniques, particularly if time was a major constraint in a research study.

The issue of time available may also determine the design and length of the questionnaire. For example, it takes less time for respondents to complete a questionnaire with closed responses than it will to complete a questionnaire with open responses that require greater effort on the part of the respondents. This is an important point for the less time it takes to complete a questionnaire, the more co-operative respondents are likely to be.

Another time-related issue is the time taken for analysis of questionnaires. Depending on the design of the questionnaire the results from self-completed surveys can be analysed quickly. However, such statements need to be seen in the context of the overall research design and effort involved in developing the questionnaires in the first instance. Questionnaires with closed questions and fixed responses can be quickly analysed, but this is less straightforward for questionnaires used in qualitative research designs that have open questions. As you will see in Chapter 10, the analysis of open questions involves a process of content analysis – a process that begins once the data are collected. If, however, the researcher is designing a questionnaire with closed questions the system of analysis is developed before the questionnaires are circulated. This can make the use of quantitatively orientated questionnaires quite an efficient way of collecting data. However, as indicated throughout this book, any approach adopted or technique used to collect data is only useful if it is the right approach for the question asked. If a quantitatively orientated, highly structured questionnaire approach is not appropriate for the research question asked, it would be a waste of time to do so.

A further advantage often credited to the use of self-administered questionnaires is that the format offers respondents anonymity. In replying to an anonymous questionnaire the respondent may be more likely to give an honest answer if he or she is confident that no one will know who has made that particular response. This is particularly so if the subject of the research study is a sensitive one.

These are some of the positive aspects related to the use of self-administered questionnaires as a research technique. As with all things, however, there are two sides to the story and some of the disadvantages may well outweigh the advantages in determining the research method used.

Disadvantages of self-administered questionnaires

Although the information so far has seemed to be in favour of utilising a self-administered questionnaire there are several major disadvantages that may be sufficient to persuade the researcher to seek an alternative approach.

The first problem is that, as noted earlier, a good questionnaire can be very difficult to design. A poorly designed questionnaire will yield only poor results. It is important to note that it is very difficult to write questions that do not introduce the risk of bias into the study. For example, the nurse wishing to ask patients about their views of treatment in hospital will find it quite difficult to formulate objective, unemotive questions in relation to this emotive experience that the patient has undergone. It is not impossible to do so, but it is not easy to write unbiased questions in relation to some aspects of care giving.

The risk of *non-compliance* by respondents is another disadvantage of self-administered questionnaires. This means that respondents do not participate in the research in the way the researcher hopes they will do so. Non-compliance can be a major source of frustration for researchers who need to consider ways in which this problem can be kept to a minimum.

Reducing non-compliance

To ensure optimum return rate the researcher will need to consider ways of distributing the questionnaires. Compliance can be linked with the fact that if left to complete questionnaires in their own time respondents may simply forget to do so. It is generally acknowledged that the method of posting questionnaires is likely to result in a lower return rate than those systems which allow the researcher direct contact with the respondents.

If using postal services a 50–60 per cent response rate is generally seen as a good response, although this of course depends on the sample size and the nature of the survey. For example people are more likely to complete questionnaires on subjects that are of interest to them and, equally, are more likely to complete questionnaires if they are not too long and require little effort on their part. If this level of return is not achieved there are some strategies that can be used to increase the return rate.

The first point to consider is the way in which you approach potential respondents and ask for their help. In Chapter 4 the need to consider the ethical dimension was discussed and, in that section, it was noted that there was a need to ensure that people participating in research do so in an informed way, and the use of a letter of introduction was discussed. This letter is also important to set the scene for potential respondents, and the way in which you write this can do much towards encouraging people to respond to your questionnaire. A friendly approach, an outline to the purpose of the research and, if appropriate, some indication of where and when the research will be reported all contribute towards whether or not people will respond to your questionnaire. To realise this you have only to consider the way that you might react to a curt abrasive letter compared with a friendly, open style of approach in a letter.

Another point to consider is the inclusion of stamped addressed envelopes for return of the questionnaire as a useful tactic to reduce non-compliance. The use of computers for word processing has really helped addressing envelopes, as a computer enables us to print out address labels or envelopes with minimum effort, so this is not the time-consuming exercise it used to be. The second point is the issue of stamps for return of completed questionnaires. You cannot expect people to pay for postage if they are responding to your questionnaire. Increasingly the stamped addressed envelope is being replaced by the use of postal systems that give a code number to indicate that postage has been paid for by the 'freepost' systems. It is worth exploring the issue of these if you are going to circulate a questionnaire to a large number of people; it may be more cost effective in the long run than buying stamps and it certainly avoids the need to stick stamps on the envelopes.

At this stage you will also need to consider how long you will give respondents to complete and return the questionnaires. Generally a two to three week time span is considered sufficient. After this time you might want to send out reminder letters to respondents if questionnaires have not been returned. This frequently results in an increase in the return rate of questionnaires, but it does so at the cost of extra time and effort for the researcher.

As postal questionnaire systems can be quite costly and frustrating in trying to yield a high response rate, an alternative approach of distributing questionnaires can be used. For example, if wishing to do a survey of 100 students it may be helpful if they could be seen by the researcher in a 'group setting'. This could perhaps be arranged if the group was in university as part of their course. This would allow the researcher to deliver and collect questionnaires personally, an aspect that usually ensures a high level of compliance. This method may yield a response rate of 75–80 per cent (or higher) and this is seen as quite a good level at which to aim.

There are ethical issues associated with compliance in completing questionnaires. The offer of a reward, however small, does affect the willingness with which people will complete questionnaires. In the business world large companies undertaking research have discovered this and may, for example, offer a reward such as a gift token as a sign of 'appreciation' for participating in a study. It is recognised that human nature is such that offers of reward or 'bribe' could have a positive impact on compliance.

The researcher in health care does not have the option open to offer rewards for ethical reasons but this aspect should not go unnoted, for the principle can be applied in some areas of research. A sample of hospital patients asked to participate in a study whilst they themselves are in a vulnerable position may see refusal to participate in a research study as a factor that may affect the quality of care they receive whilst in hospital. The researcher may know full well that a refusal would be perfectly acceptable, but it is essential that they remember that they are approaching this from a position of control, unlike the patient who is in a vulnerable position and may not have good insight into the health care system and may feel that their 'reward' for helping with the research will be better care. Equally it may be thought that staff asked to participate in a research study have a choice. The staff may not see it that way if the person undertaking the research is a senior member of management. It can be seen therefore that potential problems such as these should be identified at the outset so that no undue distress is caused to people asked to participate in research studies.

One further aspect that should be considered in relation to non-compliance is that some members of the sample group choosing not to respond to the survey may not have done so randomly. For example, if a midwife researching smoking habits in pregnancy was circulating questionnaires to pregnant mothers she may be very pleased to discover that the responses indicate a general reaction against cigarette smoking. However, further analysis of the questionnaire might reveal that all the respondents were non-smokers. The pregnant mothers who smoke may have chosen not to respond to the questionnaire and consequently their views are not represented in the analysis. This aspect of non-compliance can result in a biased result.

Other disadvantages of questionnaires

Another disadvantage of self-administered questionnaires is that they are only suitable for the literate and numerate. This may sound a fairly obvious statement but it is an aspect that can very easily be overlooked.

If we apply this point to a study of clinical practitioners and patients the problem can be illustrated further. The researcher may circulate questionnaires to nurses with confidence knowing that they will be able to complete the questionnaire. However, the level of literacy in a population over which there is little control or knowledge may cause difficulties in using this technique. For a number of reasons, including dyslexia, inability to read or write English or simply poor educational opportunity, this sample may be unable to co-operate with a questionnaire approach. Consequently the researcher should use this method with caution and take every care not to cause embarrassment.

Issues related to correct completion of questionnaires should also be considered by the researcher considering potential disadvantages of the approach. Accuracy in response is not possible to check. As you will see below, pre-testing the questionnaire before use will help identify any weakness that may contribute to this but the researcher has no control over the way in which respondents ultimately choose to answer. It is hard to deal with ambiguity and if a respondent does not make his or her meaning clear the researcher is not in a position to put an interpretation on the response. It is not uncommon to read in research reports that a number of responses have not been used in the final analysis for they were 'spoiled' and so the response was not clear to the researcher.

One further aspect that should be considered in the research design is that there is a tendency in some people when faced with a questionnaire to look for the 'right' answer. This may be a result of schooling and the habits of a lifetime. Alternatively it may occur because the respondent wants to 'help' the researcher out by giving what they see as the expected response. Again good questionnaire design should help avoid this pitfall.

If you are involved in developing a questionnaire study you might find it useful to refer to the checklist in Table 9.1. You might need to refer to other sections of this book if there are any issues identified in this table that you are not sure about.

So far we have discussed the use of self-administered questionnaires. In this approach there is very little in the way of interaction between the researcher and subject. We now need to move on to other ways of collecting data in which the researcher is more actively involved with the respondent or subject of the research.

Respondents can also be asked to complete questionnaires by direct face-to-face interview with the researcher. As you will see below this has a number of advantages but can also be disadvantageous as it is quite a time-consuming approach. We will discuss this further in the context of using interviews to collect research data.

Interview techniques in data collection

Interviews are another popular way of collecting data. In contrast to the approach in which respondents are asked to complete questionnaires, the use of interviews implies the researcher will meet respondents face to face, commonly at an individual level although, as you will see below, some research approaches involve using interviews in a group setting.

Interviews can vary in structure from a very highly structured approach to one which utilises a more open approach. At one end of the scale of interview techniques the researcher using this approach would take a structured questionnaire and simply ask the questions as written and note the response. The interview is thus seen to be highly structured and provides a means of carrying out a quantitative approach to a research study. This method, although time consuming, does have some advantages.

Table 9.1 Using questionnaires in research: some considerations

---

Before developing the questionnaire
What do I want to know?
Will this be the right instrument to use to answer my question?
Who will my respondents be?
What kind of questions will I ask (developing the questionnaire)?
Are there any ethical dilemmas involved in asking these questions?
Do I have the skills required to develop a questionnaire?

Contacting the respondents
How will I contact my respondents?
Do I need permission to approach the respondents (ethical or access)?
What will I tell them about the research I am doing?
How will I tell them – do I write a letter or contact them personally?
How much information shall I give them about the study?
What will I tell the respondents about the availability of the research report?

Developing the questionnaire
What style of questions will I use?
How will I know that all variables have been addressed?
What can I do to ensure the style of presentation is good?
How will I test my questionnaire with my sample group?
How can I check my questionnaire for reliability and validity?

Administering the questionnaire
Will I send the questionnaire to individuals or use a group setting?
How will I circulate the questionnaires (deliver by hand, use postal systems)?
What length of time shall I allocate for respondents to complete the questionnaire?
Will I send a reminder letter to people who do not reply to my questionnaire?
If sending reminder letters how long will I wait before doing so?

Data analysis
How will I analyse the data?
If qualitative data is collected how will I develop the content analysis?
If quantitative data is collected what statistical tests will I use?
What do my findings mean?

Writing the report
How will I present the results in a way that will be easily understood by the reader?
Are there any issues that emerged from the questionnaire I have not considered?
What are the strengths and limitation in the research design?
What recommendations arise out of this research?

In the first instance it avoids the problem noted above of the limitation of using self-administered questionnaires for those members of the population who are not literate or numerate. Respondents would not be faced with the embarrassment of explaining that they were not able to understand the questions asked in written form. Secondly this method allows researchers to ensure that forms are completed correctly – if not they have only themselves to blame! In addition, by completing the questionnaires themselves, the researchers are on hand to make any points of clarification required by the respondent.

At the opposite end of the scale from this highly structured format the researcher may take a more 'informal' approach and ask open-ended questions that appear to be more general in nature and which allow the respondents more scope in their reply.

Researchers using this technique will sometimes describe a 'conversational approach' to this type of research interview. Information can be collected by writing down, word for word, what the respondents say. Alternatively tape recorders or video cameras can be used to capture information that is later transcribed for analysis. This reflects a qualitative approach to research.

If approaching interviews as part of a qualitative research design the overall approach and question used will to a large extent set the agenda for the style of interviewing used. For example if a researcher is undertaking an exploratory study which is perceived as being descriptive in nature, designed to answer some clearly described questions, the researcher may set a sequence of open-ended questions that will direct the research. So for example as you will see in Table 9.2, several interview questions have been set out to find out how health care workers feel about their work – in this instance the researcher is asking the question 'What do health care workers feel about working in the NHS today?'. In response to such a question the research will yield some specific responses that could be categorised quantitatively, such as where the respondent works, how long they have worked there but other questions will yield more open responses.

Table 9.2 Interview schedule

- Where do you work?
- How long have you worked there?
- What do you think about the work you are doing?
- What makes you feel good about your work?
- What makes you feel bad about your work?
- Are your feelings about work the same as they have always been?

Now if you consider the simplicity of the questions in Table 9.2 you might think it easy to develop qualitatively orientated studies that use interview approaches but as with questionnaire design a degree of rigour is required in developing the use of this approach. Overall the same principle of questionnaire design as discussed above applies to the design of an interview schedule as this is simply another form of collecting data with the same principles. Moreover, the researcher using interview techniques to gather data will usually have undergone fairly thorough preparation before using this approach to ensure that they themselves do not introduce any bias into the proceedings. The researcher should be rigorous about keeping their own views out of the interview situation. To ensure that such objectivity is achieved it is often part of the research plan for researchers to undertake a period of training in interview techniques before collecting data in this way. If more than one researcher is involved in collecting the data, as happens in larger-scale studies, all of those involved in gathering information will undergo preparation to ensure consistency in approach to their interviews.

The preparation for interviews will involve consideration of all the stages of the interview process, that is preparing for the interview, doing the interview and analysing the data. In the preparation stage the researcher needs to consider several things in addition to the overall design of the *interviews schedule* – that is the general format used to interview a subject. This may be a questionnaire if a semi-structured approach is to be taken or simply an opening statement to open the discussion with perhaps some prompting word if a more open approach is to be taken. The kinds of thing to be considered are listed in Table 9.3.

Table 9.3 Interview preparation: some considerations

Before the interview
What do I want to know?
Will this be the right instrument to use?
Who will my respondents be?
What kind of questions will I ask (developing the interview schedule)?
Are there any ethical dilemmas involved in asking these questions?
Do I have the skills required to undertake an interview?

Contacting the respondents
How will I contact my respondents?
Do I need permission to approach the respondent (ethical or access)?
What will I tell them about the research I am doing?

Arranging the interview
How will I arrange the interview?
What length of time shall I allocate for each interview?
Where will I do the interviews?
How can I make sure the environment for the interviews is right?

Collecting the data
How will I use my interview schedule?
How will I record the data – will I write it or tape record or video the interview?
Where will I get any necessary equipment from?
How will I ensure the equipment will work?
How will I analyse the data?

The interview
How will I introduce myself to my respondents?
How can I reassure them all the information will be confidential?
How will I 'break the ice' to help them relax in the interview?
What will I do if any sensitive or ethical issues emerge?
What will I do if the interviewee starts asking me questions?
How will I close the interview?
How will I arrange any follow up interviews if necessary?
What will I tell the interviewee about the availability of the research report?

After the interview – reflection
How did that interview progress?
Are there any issues that emerged from this that I have not considered?
What are the general impressions?

Table 9.3 gives a comprehensive list of the issues you need to consider when using interviews as a technique of data collection in research. It is quite long, but if you were to work through this methodically it will take you through the total process. Broadly speaking using the interview technique in data collection involves careful consideration of the design of your interview schedule noting the points discussed above in terms of questionnaire design. In addition it requires careful consideration of the whole process of data collection both in terms of arranging interview meetings and building a rapport with respondents, considering how you will collect the data and, upon completion of an interview, how you will end the proceedings.

If your interviews follow a fairly structured approach most of these stages may be relatively straightforward. However, if you are undertaking an in-depth qualitative study you may need to give greater consideration to the way in which you approach the interview meeting. Clearly good communication skills are very important here if you want people to co-operate and, if in doubt of your ability to do this you should seek advice from your supervisor about the approach you are using. Do not assume that because your job involves you in a wide range of communication strategies on a day-to-day basis that it will be the same in the interview situation for researchers. Remember that in your job you may be communicating with people to help them, but in a research interview you are asking people to help you.

Telephone interviews

An approach to individual interviewing that has become increasingly popular in recent years is the telephone interview. This is seen as having a number of advantages, not least in saving time if you wanted to interview someone who would otherwise require a long journey to meet. Thus a researcher may be able to conduct a range of telephone interviews in the same time as it takes to set up and complete one face-to-face interview if a lot of travelling were to be involved.

There are, however, some disadvantages to this approach and in health care research telephone interviews should be used with caution. Health care researchers are reviewing it as an option in studies involving patients/clients and, in the planning stage, sometimes propose telephoning people to ask if they will become involved in a research study. Members of ethics committees may not find this approach acceptable for it has been suggested that it may be seen as being coercive in 'putting patients/clients on the spot' in terms of making a decision as to whether or not to participate in a research study. To avoid this it is advised that researchers wishing to use telephone interviews should first write to potential respondents telling them about the purpose of the study and asking if they are willing to co-operate. Potential respondents can then take time to reflect on whether to respond and, if they are able to, let the researcher know when it would be convenient to telephone to complete the interview. If there is no response to the letter this should be assumed as a negative response and the patient/client should not be contacted further. The same principles should be applied to any other sample group.

Other issues include consideration of whether telephone interviews are an appropriate medium for the study you are completing. For example if you are studying a range of issues relating to poverty it is likely that a number of the people you might wish to interview are too poor to own a telephone. Linked with this is that sampling will be restricted to people who can be contacted by telephone – this may cause a weakness in the research design.

Telephone interviews lack the potential for rapport developed in face-to-face interviews and so may lack the depth of information required if, for example you were doing a quality study. Consequently, although the benefits of telephone interviews are recognised they should be used with caution.

Group interviews

There has been an increasing interest in using group interviews in health care research as a means of identifying areas of concern and exploring issues. The term commonly used to describe such groups is '*focus group interview*'. This idea, which evolved from market research, involves a group of ten to twelve people being led in a discussion on a particular topic. The subject area is focused by using a semi-structured interview schedule but participants may, as with other forms of open interview, identify other areas of concern related to the topic that will be included in the data analysis.

Whilst this is becoming a popular approach, newcomers to research should perhaps exercise caution using it for a first project as the skill required includes not only the ability to communicate and get answers to research questions as with other interview techniques, but also skills are required in group management. It can be quite difficult to manage a group and gather and record data. For this reason texts that refer to a focus group interview commonly advise two researchers to be involved in the discussion – one to lead it and one to record it. If you want to know more about this approach refer to the further reading at the end of the chapter.

Recording data in interviews

As indicated in Table 9.3, data in interviews can be recorded manually or by using audio tape recorders or video equipment. Of these the manual recording of interviews is perhaps the most difficult. If you want to test this for yourself try recording a conversation with a friend by taking notes during the conversation. However, for some research projects this is the only appropriate way and so you would need to develop the skills required to record detail in an abbreviated form and then make sure you write up your notes in full immediately after the interview.

Tape recorders are a very popular method of recording interviews as they allow you to listen to the data when you are ready. However, they are not without problems, not least the reliability of the recorder used. Many experienced interviewers will tell you of lost data because they relied on a tape recorder that did not function properly in the course of the interview. Consequently, as noted in Table 9.3, do test any equipment before you use it. For a focus group interview you could use a tape recorder that has a 360 degree zone.

Video recording has also been noted as a means of collecting data but, as with tape recording, people may not be willing to be interviewed and monitored by video as this is quite intrusive. Whilst, in economic terms, therefore, using videos is not as costly as it once was, it may not be appropriate to use them because of respondent (and researcher!) sensitivities. However, if possible, this medium of recording data has an advantage over audio recorders in that it is possible to see as well as hear the responses to given questions.

Overall, whatever technique you use to collect interview data, as with questionnaires you should consider ways of *piloting* or at least *pre-testing* your planned approaches before the main study. This should help you identify any potential pitfalls in the approach you have chosen.

Data analysis in interview data will follow the same principle as that described above for questionnaires. Quantitative and qualitative data will be analysed using the techniques described in the next chapter.

Observation as a research technique

As with the other two approaches of questionnaire and interview the first consideration when developing a research study using observation techniques is whether this is the right approach for the research question asked. As discussed in Chapter 7 some research designs require observations as an integral part of the data collection. For example, ethnographic studies rely heavily on observation techniques. However, the choice must be made with caution, depending on the research question asked. The observation method might be appropriate to watch reactions and behaviours but it is not an appropriate method to determine how people feel about a given situation.

There are a number of advantages to using observation in research studies, not least that the researcher is seeing first hand the situation that is being studied and can focus specifically on that. In observation studies the researcher has more control over collecting information and can set the parameter of how much data they will collect, knowing the responsibility for this lies with themselves rather than relying on the co-operation of a respondent.

However, in terms of managing this approach it can be more complex than other techniques of data collection for several reasons. First, whereas people might feel quite happy about filling in a questionnaire or participating in an interview, they may not be so happy about being observed in their work or everyday life. Consequently it may be more difficult to arrange access to observe in health care situations.

Linked with this are the ethical issues of observing health care practices, which are very personal, and what to do if poor practice is observed. As a health care practitioner your first response might be that if you saw poor practice you would intervene. As a researcher this would cause you more conflict since to intervene would be the change the situation you are observing and so you would not be able to use that in your study. Only you can decide if faced with such a situation, and perhaps a useful guide is to consider the distinction between poor practice and unsafe practice.

Other problems with observation techniques lie in the time required to complete the observations and the risks of observer bias. This latter point is a common phenomenon in everyday life when we all 'see what we want or expect to see' in a given situation.

Another point to consider is the *Hawthorne effect*: a phenomenon observed in research studies in which participant's behaviour changes as a result of being observed. This was discussed in Chapter 8 where the possibility of people's behaviour changing as a result of being involved in study was considered from the perspective of the *placebo effect* – the result of someone taking an interest impacting on behaviour and thus outcome of the research. Hence, when developing the techniques for data collection in observation research the researcher needs to consider these potential pitfalls.

Collecting data in observation studies

The principles of collecting data in observation studies are the same as those described above in the context of questionnaire and interview approaches to data collection. That is, the approach used can be highly structured or low in structure.

In highly structured approaches to data collection the researcher would use a checklist approach to focus the study and, in so doing, would make very specific observations. So, if for example, the researcher was observing how restful it was for patients in hospital a number of factors relating to opportunity to rest could be included in a checklist such has the extract in Figure 9.1. Here, a number of people and situations that might interfere with rest are noted and spaces created to note interruptions in time periods.

This small example from an observation checklist serves to illustrate how quantitative data can be collected using observation measures. Using this framework

	0800hrs	0830hrs	1900hrs	0930hrs	1000hrs	1030hrs
Awake (A) asleep (S)						
Nurses						
Physiotherapist						
Social worker						
Speech therapist						
Occupational therapist						
Family						
Friend						
Noise in ward						
Noise outside ward						

Figure 9.1 Example of observation checklist for observation of patient rest in hospital.

there is scope to add any other categories seen as appropriate and the degree of specificity in each row and column would be determined by the researcher. For example, it might include notes of exactly how long a nurse spent with the patient in each time period. Alternatively the time periods could be made shorter to give more details of the number of interruptions over a given time period.

To undertake observation studies using qualitative approaches the researcher uses *field notes* to record what is observed in the course of the observations. These can be considered as similar to open-ended questions as the researcher will have areas of specific interest he or she wants to observe but are open to different experiences as they emerge in the course of the observation. In due course the notes would be analysed in the same way as other forms of qualitative data discussed in the next chapter.

Consideration could be given to the use of video cameras to observe situations but, as with the use of this medium in interviews, this can cause great sensitivity as it intrudes on the personal privacy of the participants. Moreover, there are particular ethical dilemmas with this approach in health care if it encroaches on the observation of health care, and consequently if you did want to use this approach you would need to take specific advice from your local research ethics committee and health care managers before proceeding. However, this is used in a number of situations and, with the advent of closed circuit television for security in many public buildings and the television documentary 'fly on the wall series', people are perhaps more accustomed to the idea. Certainly it is of benefit in terms of being able to 'revisit the data' at a later stage to check the observations record.

Managing observation studies

As indicated above, one of the problems with observation studies are that they are very time consuming. However, the amount of time spent will depend on the approach taken to observation. If, for example the researcher is a full *observer*, the time involved in observing can be clearly measured. However, it may be appropriate for the researcher to be a *participant observer*, which implies some degree of involvement in the situation being studied. In such cases it may not be so easy to be specific about observation times as they might be absorbed into other activities. For example, if a nurse was doing a small-scale participant observation study of how a specific treatment regime was carried out, he or she might do this in the course of his or her normal duties, stopping to observe the episodes of care as they occurred.

To complete the observation the researcher needs to make a specific schedule of observation periods that will vary depending on the nature of the subject being studied. For example if monitoring the rest patterns of patients as indicated in the example above it would be advisable to observe this over a twenty-four hour period, therefore observation sessions should be plotted out over that time. Failure to do this in such a study would not give a good indication of the totality of the rest opportunity available. In contrast, if the observation study was only focused on the physiotherapy the patient was receiving, there would be little value in observing when the physiotherapist was not there. Thus, the two types of sampling techniques referred to in observation study are *time sampling* in the first example and *event sampling* in the second example.

Whatever approach is taken there is also a need to consider the length of the time spent observing. Whilst you may feel that your working life involves a lot of observation and so you could spend a whole working day doing this, in reality this is not so. In normal life, although observing the people you care for, there are other factors that will distract you during the course of the day. If, however, you are just observing you may not be able to keep your concentration. Only you will know how long you can do this – you could try it out in your pilot test. Generally speaking, episodes of two to four hours are sufficient for observation periods and you should have a break after that.

If you are going to use an observation approach to a study you might want to refer to the checklist in Table 9.4. You might need to refer to other sections of this book if there are any issues identified in this table that you are not sure about.

Table 9.4 Observation studies preparation: some considerations

Planning the observation
What do I want to know?
Is this the right way to collect data to answer my questions?
Who will I observe?
Where will I do the observations?
What kind of things will I observe?
Are there any specific ethical issues involved or that may emerge out of this study?
How will I get ethical approval to proceed?
How will I gain access to the research site?
Do I have the skills required to do an observation study?

Arranging the observation
How will I arrange the observation?
What kind of sampling will I use – time sampling or event sampling?
What length of time shall I allocate to each observation?
Do I need further permission to observe individuals (patients/clients/relatives/staff)?
What will I tell the people I am observing about what I am doing?

Collecting the data
How will I structure my observations – schedule or field notes?
How will I record the data? (Are videos a possibility?)
How will I analyse the data?
How will I introduce myself to the people I am observing?
How can I reassure them all the information will be confidential?
What will I do if any sensitive or ethical issues emerge?
What will I do if the people I am observing start asking me questions?

Completing observations
How will I leave the area in which I am observing?
How will I arrange to follow up the people I am observing (if appropriate)?
What will I tell the people I observed about the availability of the research report?

After the observation – reflection
How did that observation progress?
Are there any issues that emerged from this that I have not considered?
What are the general impressions?

Other techniques of data collection

The three types of data collection noted above (questionnaire, interviews and observation) are the major techniques used in health care research. However, there are other resources available to researchers that do not fall neatly into the techniques described. For example researchers may access data from diaries or other forms of records. To do this they can use qualitative or quantitative approaches. For example if using a diary it would be appropriate to use qualitative techniques of data analysis described in the next chapter. If using medical records to determine the ranges of diagnostic categories treated by a community health care team over the last year, a more structured, quantitatively orientated checklist would be appropriate. Other forms of data used by members of the health care team include physiological measures, for example if the physiotherapist is measuring mobility or if the doctor is measuring the blood level of a new drug.

Whatever form of data is used the researcher will consider ways in which reliability and validity can be ensured in terms of the data collected.

Reliability and validity

Reliability in research instruments reflects the degree to which an instrument used for data collection provides consistent responses when used under similar conditions. Validity is the extent to which the instrument measures what is supposed to be measured. Because of this distinction it should be noted that a researcher using quantitative approaches will endeavour to ensure that any structured technique of data collection used will be reliable. Much of the effort involved in developing a questionnaire for example is to address this issue. Researchers using quantitative approaches will also endeavour to ensure that techniques of data collection are valid and will spend a lot of time refining their questionnaire to ensure this is so. On the other hand, researchers using some qualitative methods will know from the outset that they are not going to get a 'consistent response' to the questions they ask – open-ended questions can yield such a range of responses. However, in focusing the study on the individual perspective qualitative researchers may claim their studies are more valid than quantitative studies which to varying extents decontextualise the subject being researched.

Reliability

There are three ways that are commonly used to test reliability and to illustrate this the development of questionnaires will be considered. The first of these is known as the *test–retest* approach. This determines the degree of consistency when individual responses are compared on two separate occasions. To do this you would ask respondents to complete the first draft of your questionnaire. You would then administer the questionnaire on a second occasion, usually several weeks after the first completion to ensure respondents do not remember what they said on the first occasion. If the results from each individual respondent were the same on the two occasions you may conclude that you are getting a consistent response to your questions under similar conditions. If the results were not consistent you would need to reconsider the design of your questions.

Another way of doing this is to complete a *parallel form* test which measures the degree of consistency when individuals respond to two forms of the same instrument. If, for example, you decide to develop a questionnaire for stress and want to test how reliable it is, you could test it against another stress questionnaire that has already been shown to be reliable and valid and compare the results. If your questionnaire was reliable it should indicate the same level of stress as the other scale.

Questionnaires can also be examined for reliability in the context of *internal consistency*. This is a measure of the degree of agreement in response between items that are examining different aspects of similar issues. So, for example, if you asked the question whether your respondents smoked and they answered 'no' you would not then expect them to indicate later that they smoked thirty cigarettes a day in another question.

These techniques lend themselves more readily to highly structured approaches to data collection but the principle can be adapted for other techniques. For example, open questions should yield the same response from respondents if asked on more than one occasion.

Researchers using observation to collect data also need to consider whether their methods are reliable. They can check this by sharing some observations with a colleague to determine if they are seeing and recording the same phenomenon. Clearly this is easier to do if developing a quantitative study as the same principles discussed above apply.

Validity

Validity has three dimensions. The first, *face validity*, is a judgement of whether on the 'face of it' the research instrument appears to measure what it is supposed to measure. *Content validity* is the term used to indicate how well content appears to measure what it is supposed to measure. For example if you wanted to test intelligence, are the questions doing that? *Construct validity* focuses on the theoretical base of the questionnaire and asks the questions of whether the theory underlying the test is measured. For example you may have noted that personality tests often draw on a range of issues to measure dimensions of personality. Finally *criterion-related validity* questions how well the test relates to other external measures of the same phenomenon. This is similar to the point made above under the heading of reliability – if testing stress using a new questionnaire the outcome should be the same in the validated tool and the new tool, i.e. both should indicate stress or both should indicate no stress.

ACTIVITY _____

- Refer to the topic you identified that you might like to research (activity in Chapter 3). In the last chapter you noted whether this was a qualitative or a quantitative orientation.
- Now, in the context of that decision consider which technique it would be best to use to collect data.
- Now list the reasons why you think this technique is the best approach for you.
- List the reasons why the other approaches may be inappropriate.

Summary

This chapter has explored some of the research techniques available and considered some of the advantages and disadvantages of collecting information by using questionnaires, interviews and observational techniques. In recognition of the limited space available to explore all of these issues in depth, readers wishing to use these approaches when undertaking research studies are recommended to consult the further reading.

Further reading

Bell, J. (1993) *Doing Your Research Project? A Guide for First Time Researchers in Education and the Social Sciences*, Open University Press, Buckingham.

Cormack, D.F.S. (1991) *The Research Process in Nursing*, 2nd edn, Blackwell Scientific, Oxford, Chs 20–24.

Fowler, F.J. (1993) *Survey Research Methods*, 2nd edn, Sage, London.

Moser, C.A. and Kalton, G. (1971) *Survey Methods in Social Investigation*, Heinemann Educational, London.

Oppenheim, A.N. (1992) *Questionnaire Design and Attitude Measurement*, Heinemann Educational, London.

Stone, D.H. (1995) 'Design a questionnaire', *British Medical Journal*, vol. 307, pp. 1264–1266.

See also the following journals: *Nurse Researcher*, 'Observation', vol. 2, no. 2, December (1994); 'Interviewing technique', vol. 1, no. 3, March (1994); 'Outcome measures in quantitative research', vol. 2, no. 4, June (1995).

10 Analysing and presenting research data

This chapter will examine the principles of data analysis and explore ways in which research data can be presented. It will serve as a broad introduction to the topic rather than a 'how to do it guide'. Readers who wish to develop their skills in data analysis are referred to the further reading at the end of the chapter. The chapter will explore three main areas:

1. Data analysis in qualitative research designs.
2. Data analysis in quantitative research designs.
3. Presenting research data.

Data analysis in qualitative research designs

As indicated in Chapter 7, qualitative research designs involve collecting data in words. Those words might be generated by a respondent as a result of an interview, or by a researcher making notes as part of his or her field work in a study involving observation. Other forms of data in words can be generated by referring to records or diaries that contribute to the phenomenon being studied. However data are collected, the process of analysis in qualitative research designs is known as content analysis.

Content analysis

Content analysis involves the researcher in analysing the words generated through data collection. This involves looking closely for patterns or themes that recur in the data to provide an explanation of what was discovered through the research.

The nature of the data the researcher is working with will influence the level of complexity of the process of content analysis. This will vary depending on the overall research design adopted and the techniques used to collect data. For example if a researcher uses a descriptive qualitative research design to develop a questionnaire with several open questions that will be self-completed by the respondents, the scope of reply will be limited by the space available on the page.

For example a researcher examining quality of care issues might ask the respondent to '*Identify what you feel were the positive aspects of your experience in this unit*'. Such a question will generate a limited response if given in questionnaire format. This means that in response to each question the researcher might only need to analyse a few lines of responses. This can be contrasted with the volume of words that could be generated by the researcher asking the same question verbally and using prompts to encourage the respondent to elaborate on the issues raised.

Analysing qualitative data

However data are collected the first step in data analysis is to make the data readily accessible for analysis. The second step is to 'reduce' the data into a manageable format and the third is, on the basis of the previous two steps, to draw conclusions about the research findings. The starting point in the analysis is therefore to consider how to make the data *accessible*. In the example above, the researcher using the questionnaire has the data readily available in written form. A researcher using tape recorded interviews, however, needs to consider how to make the data more accessible. Whilst it is feasible to access data generated by interview by listening to it repeatedly, this can be very time consuming and does not create a medium whereby others can check the·interpretation of the data. Consequently it is the convention for researchers using this approach to make the data accessible by transcribing it into a written format for analysis. Any transcription of data in research can be done manually but the advent of computer technology has resulted in a number of authors suggesting that qualitative data be transcribed to a word processing package for this can help the subsequent analysis process.

Once the data are transcribed the next step in the process of analysis is to *reduce* the data by drawing out words, phrases or general statements that can be identified as common patterns or themes in the data. This can be quite a cumbersome process. It can involves either a sentence-by-sentence analysis in which general ideas, or themes are drawn from the data. Alternatively a word-by-word analysis enables the researcher to draw out words that commonly recur in the data and from this to develop a picture of what is happening.

There are advantages and disadvantages to each approach and, as with other forms of data analysis, it is important that you consider the extent to which you wish to analyse your data before you start your research. To some extent this may be determined by the way in which the data are collected. If data are collected by questionnaire, for example, the range of qualitative data collected might be quite limited in terms of the number of words generated by respondents and so relatively easy to analyse on a word-by-word basis. In contrast, interview data can be quite cumbersome and a word-by-word analysis will take a lot longer. Sometimes, therefore, researchers who have undertaken in-depth interviews will undertake a process of thematic analysis first, to look for common patterns in sentences and paragraphs before undertaking a more detailed word-by-word approach. This enables them to exclude any data that are not directly relevant to the research topic and makes the data more manageable. This is an important point, for qualitative researchers commonly note that the nature of data collection through qualitative techniques will commonly yield data that are superfluous to the phenomenon being studied. It is important to exclude these data as soon as possible so that they do not cloud the interpretation and conclusions.

As the data analysis proceeds the researcher begins to organise the data by using codes to indicate the relevance of the reduced data. These codes start out in broad categories. So, for example in response to the question: '*Identify what you feel were the positive aspects of your experience in this unit*', several respondents might have noted 'communication' as an issue and used examples to illustrate this. In this instance the researcher might use a code to indicate that communication was a common theme and would place the code number allocated to this alongside every piece of information relating to communication. This pattern would continue with each theme identified until no new themes emerge for analysis. This is known as the point of 'saturation' of the data.

Some researchers may simply stop at this point and, having identified categories or themes, note the frequency with which they occur. Some research texts refer to this notion and suggest that in counting the frequency of occurrences of particular statement the researcher is in fact measuring qualitative data, a term sometimes referred to as 'quantifying qualitative data'. Whilst this may be criticised by some qualitative researchers it really comes back to the point of undertaking a qualitative approach to the research in the first place. If, as indicated in Chapter 7, a qualitative approach was undertaken to explore and describe a situation, this is not unacceptable as the purpose of the research may simply be to identify themes in the data. In the example above it might be useful to indicate how frequently an issue such as communication was mentioned as it could be a clear indicator of the experience if noted by most respondents. However, this may not be sufficient if using some of the other approaches to qualitative research discussed in Chapter 7 as this type of analysis does not capture the 'richness' of the data.

The researcher who wished to undertake a more complex analysis will move on to another level of analysis once the initial codes have been identified. At this point it is usual to start combining themes and ideas that have emerged in the first round of data analysis. For example, communication might be submerged under a theme labelled 'relationships'.

This level of analysis is a more complex process, beyond the scope of this introductory text; if you wish to consider it further, refer to the further reading at the end of the chapter.

The final step in the analysis stage of qualitative research design is *drawing conclusions* from the data. If the researcher has 'quantified' the data into categories it may be relatively easy to draw conclusions by noting the frequency with which some aspects relating to the phenomenon being studied were identified and conclusions on what may be seen in terms of patterns of responses noted. However, with most qualitative research the stage of drawing conclusions is usually more complex than this and is commonly based on the second or third round of analysis which has already involved some interpretation in the identification and refinement of themes or categories. At this stage the researcher will be asking questions such as:

'What does this mean?'

'What is the data telling me about phenomena I am studying?'

'Have I been fair in my interpretation of the data?'

'If others see my interpretation will they agree with my interpretation?'

'Are the findings meaningful?'

In other words the researcher is asking questions related to the reliability and validity of the data collection and analysis. As indicated in Chapter 9 reliability refers to consistency in data collection and this is difficult to achieve in qualitative research designs. If, for example, you were asking open interview questions you would not expect each respondent to answer in the same way; thus you could not say your interview schedule was producing reliable responses. In contrast, validity in qualitative research designs is said to be high as it 'measures what it is supposed to measure' in asking respondents to respond in their own words. Some authors suggest that it is therefore inappropriate to consider reliability in qualitative research designs. In so doing they suggest other criteria such as credibility of the data. Researchers completing qualitative studies commonly endeavour to check the credibility or affirm the validity of their findings by returning their analysis of the data to the subjects of the study to ask them to check if it sounds 'true' to them.

Data analysis in quantitative research designs

As indicated earlier in this text research designs that are classified as quantitative generate data that can be analysed numerically. To do this researchers use statistics. The purpose of statistics is to summarise data, so helping researchers analyse data and enabling them to communicate the findings in a form that represents shared understanding between the researcher and the reader. Statistics, therefore, can be seen as a type of shorthand, giving a synopsis of the data collected in a research study rather than by writing every detail in long hand.

Although there are a large number of people in society who have no difficulty manipulating facts and figures, for many newcomers to research one of the most daunting challenges is that of understanding the use of statistics. The language can serve to confuse if the reader is not familiar with the terminology used in statistics and consequently there can be a tendency to be suspicious of information presented in statistical form. As one of the reasons for using statistics is to present information in a form that is easy to read and understand, any negative reaction to the subject should be overcome as quickly as possible. Some insight into statistics should serve to demystify the subject and make it seem less complex.

Types of statistical test

As noted above anyone undertaking a research study must decide when they are developing a study what it is they want to measure and how they will measure it. This is important, for the way in which statistics are used will vary depending on the research design. If, for example, a researcher was undertaking a descriptive study and collecting quantitative data, let us say by using a questionnaire with forced choice response (see Chapter 9), the number and range of responses can be summarised by using descriptive statistics. *Descriptive statistics* is the type of statistics used to describe and summarise data. It offers a means by which the researcher can describe the results concisely in terms of their most important features.

Experimental research is an approach which looks for cause and effect between variables. In this case researchers will use the statistical test to help them identify whether the independent variable has caused an effect on the dependent variable. In this case the researcher will use the statistical tests to infer meaning from the data and so the tests used in experimental design are known as *inferential statistics*. As the title implies, inferential statistics may be used to 'infer' things about a population from the sample that has been studied. Unlike descriptive statistics in which the information to be analysed is readily available and pertaining to a clearly defined situation, inferential statistics are used when there is a wish to generalise research findings from a sample of a given population to the whole of that population. The term used to describe this is statistical inference.

If the researcher was using a correlational research design and looking for relationships between variables in the data the researcher may use *correlational statistical tests*.

We will consider briefly below how researchers decide which statistical test is appropriate for their study.

Choosing statistical tests

The reliability of the results obtained through analysis will depend, in the first instance, on the quality of the research instruments and the quality of the data collection. It is only when you are confident that your techniques of collecting quantifiable data are reliable and valid that you should turn to the statistical tests available to help you in your analysis.

One of the difficulties facing newcomers to research is deciding which statistical test they should use for the research. This is the point at which the background knowledge of research design that has been covered so far in this text is used to help in decision making as, overall, the type of test you use will be that deemed appropriate to the research design as indicated in Figure 10.1. For example, under the descriptive design heading measures of central tendency and measures of dispersion are cited. In the correlational design column two types of correlational test, the Spearman test and the Pearson test are noted. In the experimental column two categories of test,

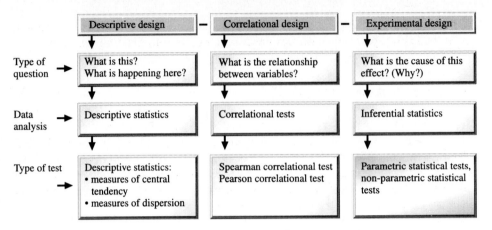

Figure 10.1 Research design and statistical tests.

namely parametric and non-parametric tests, are noted. Each of these will be explored below.

Descriptive statistics

When using statistics the researcher is trying to make sense of the information available to them and to present it in some form that will be meaningful to others. As indicated above, statistics are a way of summarising data. There are many ways in which this can be done in everyday working life and, probably without thinking about it very much you will have become quite accomplished at working with descriptive statistics in your work or studies.

Measurements used in descriptive statistics

Research studies utilising quantitative techniques collect data that can be subject to some form of numerical measurement as described below.

Percentages

At a fairly simple level the use of percentages is a very useful way of analysing data as it indicates patterns in data at a simple level. For example, if a class of 100 students took an exam and of these 84 were successful, the pass rate could be described as 84 per cent. Use of percentages also offers quite a simple way of comparing two groups of unequal size. If out of a second group of 67 students, 41 students had passed the exam, the pass rate will be 61 per cent. The first group of students can therefore be seen to have a better pass rate than the second. In descriptive research design, quantifiable data percentage ratings are commonly used to illustrate findings.

Measures of central tendency

There are several other measures which are commonly used in descriptive statistics. The use of these measures helps to interpret the meaning behind a set of results and offers a useful way of presenting results in a summarised form. *Measures of central tendency* represent the results in terms of the most common features. These measures describe the 'central' scores in the distribution of a set of figures. Three commonly used measures are the mean, median and mode.

Mean

The mean is another word for the average. It is represented by the symbol $\bar{x}$ or the letter m and is the sum of the observations noted divided by the total number of observations. So, for example, if you had collected data to indicate the number of people who had used your service over the last ten days you would calculate the total number of treatments and divide by 10 to find the mean. Using this, the mean number of clients from the list in Table 10.1 is 15.

Table 10.1 Example of the mean: number of clients treated over ten days

Day 1	13
Day 2	10
Day 3	15
Day 4	21
Day 5	14
Day 6	16
Day 7	18
Day 8	18
Day 9	13
Day 10	12
Total	**150** ($\bar{x} = 15$)

Of the three measures of central tendency the mean is the most commonly used statistic for it is more reliable and accurate than the others. This is because the mean depends on the value of every score and alteration in one score will have an impact on the mean. The disadvantage of using the mean, however, also lies in this factor since a fairly radical change in just one score may have a dramatic effect on the mean.

The mean does not give any information about the spread or distribution of scores. For example, if the number of patients admitted to a hospital ward (Table 10.2) in June was reduced to 4, and the number of admissions in February was increased to 53 the mean score would remain at 20. However, the distribution of scores has changed in those months.

Table 10.2 Number of patients admitted to hospital wards in a twelve month period

Month	Number of patients
January	26
February	35
March	15
April	29
May	16
June	22
July	10
August	11
September	14
October	16
November	18
December	28
Total	**240** ($\bar{x} = 20$)

Median

The *median* represents a score that is the midpoint in a set of results. If the total number of observations is arranged from the smallest to the largest, the median represents what may be seen as the midpoint in that half the scores are larger than and half are less than the median. For example in the figures noted in a set of observations below, the median is 27 as this is the figure that falls midway in the observations:

$$11 \quad 20 \quad 23 \quad 27 \quad 30 \quad 33 \quad 35$$

If the number of observations noted equals an even number then the median is said to represent the midpoint between the two middle scores. For example, in Table 10.2 there are twelve observations which have been listed in numerical order as follows:

$$10 \quad 11 \quad 14 \quad 15 \quad 16 \quad 16 \quad 18 \quad 22 \quad 26 \quad 28 \quad 29 \quad 35$$

In this case the two middle scores are 16 and 18. To find the median you need to calculate the mean for the middle figures, so 16 + 18 divided by 2 gives a median of 17.

One of the problems in using the median is that a given set of figures could be altered quite radically and yet the median would remain the same. For example, in the numbers of patients noted in Table 10.2, the highest number is 35. If this was changed to 350, the median would still remain the same. (It should be noted that this feature can, however, sometimes make the median more useful than the mean since a score of 35 is more representative of the data than the mean which would change to 46.25.) It can be seen therefore that the disadvantage of using the median is that it gives no information about the range of scores. It is unreliable and unstable as it could either be altered drastically by a single figure or not at all.

Mode

The *mode* is the expression used to describe the observation that occurs most frequently in the sample of data. In Table 10.2, when referring to the number of patients admitted, the mode can be seen to be 16. This is the number that occurs most frequently throughout the population noted and is the most common score.

As with the median, the mode is seen to be an unreliable and unstable measure for altering one figure drastically can have a major impact or no effect at all. In other words it gives no information about how data are distributed. If the number of admissions noted in Table 10.2 was increased to 60 in January and 80 in February the mode would still be 16. If the number of admissions in May and June was increased to 35 the mode would change to 35.

Measures of dispersion

The measures of central tendency have a limitation in that the mean, median and mode do not give a clear picture of how the data are spread. There is no indication as to whether the individual scores in a sample are close to the mean or are widely dispersed. This has practical implications in health care situations. For example a manager may have been given the mean number of patients/clients treated in a clinical area. Although a useful statistic, this alone may not help him or her in the deployment of staff for the number of treatments each week could change very markedly and thus have implications for manpower planning. What this manager needs to know is the range of treatments in the unit. The statistics used to indicate this are known as measures of dispersion for they are used to describe the distribution of data. Range, variance and deviation will be discussed below to illustrate the use of these measures.

Range

The *range* is a term used to describe the difference between the lowest and the highest value in a given set of figures. This is a useful measure for it indicates the degree of difference between the two. To calculate the range the smallest score is subtracted from the highest. Thus if the highest number of admissions to the ward in one week was 25 and the lowest was 2 the range would be calculated thus:

$$25 - 2 = 23$$

The range is said to be 23.

To illustrate this further let us look at the two sets of results produced by students on a health studies programme in their exams (Table 10.3). The range of grades awarded in group A indicate that one student has failed to achieve the pass grade (indicated as 50 in Table 10.3) while in group B three out of six students have failed the exam. The range for group A results is $52 - 46 = 6$. Group B range is $90 - 12 = 78$. A small range indicates a more homogenous set of data than a large range. This may be important when interpreting results. For example, an examiner comparing the range of the two sets of results would note the difference in scores between the two sets of students in the example above. However, the numbers of 6 and 78 as noted above do not mean very much on their own. There is a need to identify how the scores are distributed. To do this, *deviation* or *variance* measures are used.

Table 10.3 Examination results: students on health studies programme

	Group A			Group B
	46			12
	51			15
	50			18
	52			79
	50			90
	51			86
Total	**300 ($\bar{x} = 50$)**		**Total**	**300 ($\bar{x} = 50$)**

Pass mark = 50.

Deviation and variance

To calculate how far each set of scores deviates from the mean, the mean is subtracted from each score thus indicating the position of each score relative to the mean. If you do this with the results from students in groups A and B you will note the degree of deviation from the mean in both groups. Group A is obviously much closer to the mean (Table 10.4).

Table 10.4 Deviation from the mean where $\bar{x} = 50$

Group A	Group B
46–50 = −4	10–50 = −40
51–50 = +1	12–50 = −38
50–50 = 0	15–50 = −35
52–50 = +2	89–50 = +39
50–50 = 0	90–50 = +40
51–50 = +1	86–50 = +36

Although the information in Table 10.4 gives a useful indicator of the deviation from the mean by the calculation of every score, it can result in a presentation of data that appears complex and cumbersome. Consequently it might be useful to group data to indicate the degree of variance for the group. This can be done by squaring each deviation score and totalling the products to achieve the *variance*. Thus the results from the students in group A can be computed:

$$(-4)^2 + (1)^2 + (0)^2 + (2)^2 + (0)^2 + (1)^2 = 16 + 1 + 0 + 4 + 0 + 1 = 22$$

The variance figure represents the total variance of a set of scores. The variance of a set of scores indicates how dispersed or varied the scores are. The smaller the variance, the more similar the scores. The greater the variance score, the more disparate the results. To illustrate this point it may be useful for you to calculate the variance score for the students in group B and to compare the result with that noted above for group A students.

This type of calculation is an integral part of several statistical tests that you may need to do when developing your own research work and so it is a useful concept to understand at this stage as you begin to learn about research.

Standard deviation (SD)

Another calculation that is commonly used in research is the standard deviation. This is the most important of the measures of dispersion for it represents the average or standard degree of deviation in a set of scores rather than the total degree of variation. If the amount of dispersion is large (as with the students in group B) so the standard deviation will have a greater numerical value.

The formula used to describe the standard deviation can look complex to the newcomer but, if broken down into component parts, is not so difficult to understand. If you can see how one formula is presented then it is easier to apply the principles when faced with other statistical tests. The formula is:

$$SD = \sqrt{\frac{\Sigma(x - \bar{x})^2}{n}}$$

This means:

SD = standard deviation (sometimes written as σ),

$\sqrt{}$ = square root of all the calculations under the symbol. (NB The square root of a number x = the number which when multiplied by itself gives x, e.g. square root of 9 = 3 as $3 \times 3 = 9$),

x = individual score,

x^2 = squared number multiplied by itself (this is the variance score described above),

$\bar{x}$ = mean score,

Σ = the total sum,

n = total number of scores in the sample group. (The symbol $n - 1$ is used in inferential statistics when inferring information about the population from which the sample was taken, n is used when the SD from the sample only is used.)

Normal distribution

Within any set of results researchers are concerned with whether the distribution of the data represents a '*normal distribution*'. This is an important concept for statistical purposes and it is one that is demonstrated visually to demonstrate the point.

A 'normal' distribution could be identified by the following example. If a large random sample of women living in the United Kingdom had their height measured and the results were plotted on a graph it is likely that the pattern that emerged on the graph would be a 'bell shape'. This bell-shaped pattern is described as a normal distribution curve. It is useful in statistical terms for it allows some degree of prediction to be made about the data gathered. In addition some of the tests undertaken in inferential statistics rely on an assumption of normal distribution of data (see Figure 10.2).

It may be anticipated that if a *random sample* was selected, that the majority of women would be about the same height, a few would be short and a few tall. If you

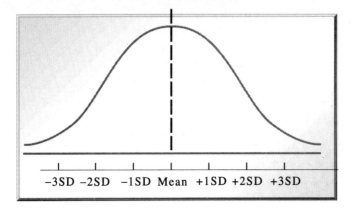

Figure 10.2 Normal distribution curve.

were to undertake such a survey and found that the distribution of heights was 'normal' you could calculate the mean, median and mode and you would find them to be the same.

It can be noted that the standard deviation is marked on the diagram (Figure 10.2) and a fixed percentage of scores in a set of normally distributed data fall within each standard deviation. In a normally distributed set of data, 34 per cent of observations lie within one standard deviation either side of the mean, therefore 68 per cent will always fall in this range. It is on this basis that the curve is useful in predicting what percentage of a population will fall into a given range.

It should be noted that not all data are normally distributed and other terms may be given to describe the pattern that emerges when results are plotted on a graph. A *skewed* distribution can be described as a negative or positive pattern. Figures 10.3 and 10.4 show this. Such skewed patterns may occur if the data collected were not 'normal', for example, if a large number of women had been shown to be tall or a large number were seen to be small. In such situations where there is a skewed pattern in the data collection the median might be a more useful measure than the mean.

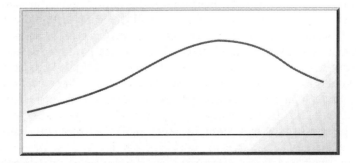

Figure 10.3 Negative skew.

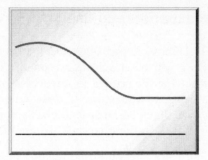

Figure 10.4 Positive skew.

Other types of pattern can occur if data are plotted in graph form; for example, reference may be made to *bi-modal* curves or *J-shaped* curves. To find out more about these refer to the further reading at the end of the chapter. It is useful to appreciate these terms for they may be used in research texts when describing the range of results obtained in a study.

Inferential statistical tests

Inferential statistical tests are used to test a *hypothesis*. When developing the statistical test you will write a *null hypothesis* (see Chapter 8). If the results from the statistical tests are said to be *significant* this means that the null hypothesis is rejected and the hypothesis is therefore accepted. If the results are not significant then the null hypothesis is accepted. So, you need to understand what is meant by significance in research.

Significance

Significance is a statistical term for a result that tells you the *probability* of an error occurring in the results of a study. Because it refers to probability the significance is usually indicated by referring to probability using the letter p. So, for example you might see in a research report that the researcher has concluded that the results of a set of tests are significant with $p = 0.05$. This indicates that the results show there is a 5 per cent chance that the results of the research study may be due to random error or chance rather than to the effect of the independent variable on the dependent variable as stated in the hypothesis. In other words, 5 cases in 100 might show a result due to error or chance. In health care research, a significance level of 5 per cent ($p = 0.05$) is the level that is set for much of the research you will read. This may differ in research studies that involve any potential threat to health, as a lower level of error or risk may be required. For example, in clinical drug trials the significance level may be set at 1 per cent ($p = 0.01$).

Statistical tests in experimental design

If you refer to Figure 10.1 above it was suggested that in experimental design the kind of test you might use will be classed as parametric or non-parametric tests. *Parametric tests* must meet specific criteria in terms of sampling, the nature of the data collected and the range of responses. If these criteria cannot be met then *non-parametric tests* are used. Each parametric test has a non-parametric equivalent.

The conditions required for parametric tests to be used include the following:

1. The data collected must use interval/ratio measures (see Chapter 9).
2. The data must be approximately normally distributed.
3. The range of the data corresponding to each of the groups of subjects should be fairly similar.
4. The subjects should be selected at random (see Chapter 6).

Using this list you can see, for example, that parametric tests should not be used in studies collecting nominal data or in studies where it is not possible to select a random sample.

The choice of statistical test that is appropriate for your study will depend on the overall research design you have adopted. As indicated, the type of data collected is important as different tests will be used for nominal, for ordinal data or interval/ratio data. To help the researcher in this, each test has specific criteria attached to it and some texts use 'decision charts' to help researchers make their decisions. A small extract of such a decision chart has been included in Figure 10.5.

As you see in Figure 10.5, each question prompts you towards the next step of deciding which statistical test to use. So, if you had used a *matched subject design* (see Chapter 8) that met the criteria for a parametric test, the test you would do is a related *t* test. In contrast if you had used a *different subject design* which did not meet the criteria for a parametric test you would use a non-parametric test, the Mann–Whitney *U* test. If you refer to the research tests identified in the further reading section at the end of this chapter they will generally carry specific guidelines such as this to lead you to the appropriate statistical test.

Statistical tests in correlational design

You will remember from Chapter 8 that correlational research studies start with a hypothesis that proposes a relationship between two variables. What we want to know in such tests is the nature of the relationship. To help in this there are two important concepts that you need to understand: positive and negative correlation. If, as a result of statistical analysis, a *positive correlation* is identified this indicates that an *increase* in the score of one variable is associated with an *increase* in the score of the other variable. In contrast, if a set of results indicated a negative correlation, an *increase* in one variable is associated with a *decrease* in the other.

For example look at Table 10.5 which indicates the hours spent on physiotherapy for a sports injury alongside the number of days taken for recovery. In this example

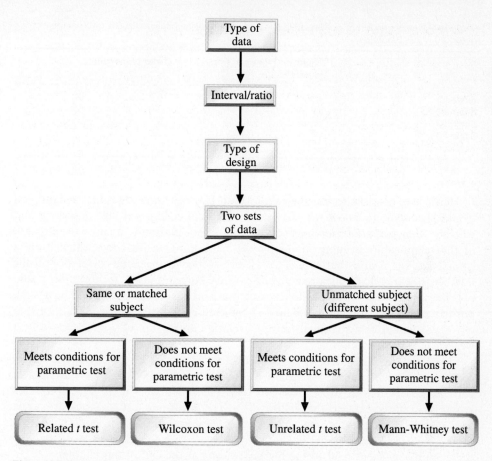

Figure 10.5 Extract from a statistical decision-making flow chart.

Table 10.5 Number of hours of physiotherapy and recovery rate

	Number of hours of physiotherapy	Speed of recovery in days
Subject 1	12	5
Subject 2	11	6
Subject 3	10	7
Subject 4	9	8
Subject 5	7	9

there is a negative correlation as the greater the number of hours, the less the number of days to recovery. In contrast if you look at Table 10.6 you will see a positive correlation in that the greater the number of hours spent on physiotherapy, the greater the degree of mobility as measured on a ten-point scale.

Table 10.6 Number of hours of physiotherapy compared with mobility measured on a ten-point scale (where 10 = good mobility)

	Number of hours of physiotherapy	Level of mobility
Subject 1	12	10
Subject 2	11	9
Subject 3	10	8
Subject 4	9	7
Subject 5	7	6

Whilst it is possible to see the relationship between these two sets of data, you would also want to know the *strength* of the relationship you are observing and whether what you are observing is *significant*. In correlational research the strength of the relationship is summed up by the final sum reached once calculation is completed. The nearer that sum is to $+1$ or -1 the stronger the correlation. If the number is near $+1$ it indicates a strong positive correlation, so, for example, a sum of 0.986 would be a strong positive correlation and a sum of 0.345 would be a weak positive correlation. A number near -1 indicates a negative correlation, so a sum of -0.988 would be a strong negative correlation and a sum of -0.321 would be a weak negative correlation.

The statistical tests used in correlation design is referred to as the *correlation coefficient* which measures the extent of the relationship between two variables in correlational statistical tests. (The two tests referred to in Figure 10.1 above are examples of statistical tests that indicate this. The Spearman test is a non-parametric test and the Pearson test is a parametric test.) The correlation coefficient is a measure of *how well two variables are related*. If you want to know how to work out the correlation coefficient refer to the further reading at the end of this chapter.

Computers and research

Before we leave the subject of data analysis in research it should be noted briefly that computers are a very useful resource to researchers planning to undertake statistical tests. Many computer firms produce software packs that can be used to analyse research data. These have proved to be a big time saver for anyone wishing to do statistical testing in research. If the researcher wishes to take advantage of such packages he or she should consider this issue early in the planning stage of the study so that the research design matches the facilities available for analysis. The rate of development of computer technology is such that it advisable to ask for help from experts for they will be able to advise on the most recent developments. Health care workers wishing to use computers to help analyse research findings could seek advice from academic staff in universities or from local advisors available through NHS research centres.

Presenting research data

There are several ways in which researchers may present their data in summarised form. These include using tables, graphs, histograms and pie charts.

Tables

One of the commonest means of presenting numerical information is to use tables to summarise findings. Tables should be clearly labelled so that the reader knows the purpose without having to scour the text for clarification. In addition they should be as simple as possible since rows and rows of figures can be very difficult for the reader to interpret. It is suggested in some statistical texts that it is better to have two simple tables than a single, complex one.

If Table 10.7 is reviewed it can be seen that it indicates how the total number of people over the age of 75 years has risen in a village community over the past ten years. The table also distinguishes the number of men and women represented in that group. Such data might be useful when planning service provision for this group of potential clients.

Table 10.7 Number of people over 75 years living in Groom

Year	Male	Female	Total
1987	15	14	29
1988	14	18	32
1989	14	19	33
1990	13	22	35
1991	13	19	32
1992	15	25	40
1993	17	22	39
1994	19	21	40
1995	25	30	55
1996	29	34	63
Total	174	224	398

Table 10.8 gives an indication of seasonal trends in the types of admissions in that medical ward area. You can see there are far more admissions with bronchitis in the winter months. Another point that is useful to note at this stage is that a symbol commonly used to identify the total number of individuals or objects studied is n. Hence in Table 10.8 the expression '$n = 967$' indicates that the total sample for this study is 967 people. Abbreviations such as this allow tables to carry a lot of relevant information in a very limited space.

Table 10.8 Diagnostic categories of admissions to a hospital ward during a twelve month period ($n = 967$)

Month	Bronchitis	Cardiac	Neurological	Other	Total
January	30	15	15	20	80
February	36	26	20	13	95
March	36	10	8	41	95
April	28	30	12	18	88
May	20	20	15	25	80
June	20	15	13	22	70
July	20	20	18	8	66
August	10	18	20	20	68
September	10	15	15	30	70
October	12	20	20	18	70
November	28	15	12	32	87
December	30	22	26	20	98
Total	**280 (29%)**	**226 (23%)**	**194 (20%)**	**267 (28%)**	**967 (100%)**

The use of percentages in this table gives additional meaning to the results. For example, the fact that 280 patients admitted with bronchitis represents 29% of the 967 patients admitted to the ward may be quite an important point for mangers of health care planning to meet the needs for different groups of patients.

The advantage to the researcher, and subsequently the reader, of presenting data in a numerical form in tables is that it offers a type of shorthand, a very simple means of summarising a series of recordings or observations. The information in Tables 10.7 and 10.8 can be quickly reviewed and trends identified.

The researcher presenting any results from a study needs to have in mind the potential preferences of the reader when writing the report. There are some people who are able to interpret numerical information very quickly whilst others need the implications spelt out very clearly. In the majority of research reports note has been taken of this. Although there may be a scattering of tables of numerical values the interpretation of these results is spelt out in clear terms alongside. Tables are frequently used simply to support the points made in the written report.

There are several other ways in which the researcher can present data to make it easier for the reader to review by summarising key points. Of these the most commonly used are *graphs, histograms, bar charts* and *pie charts*.

Graphs

The use of *graphs* is familiar to all health care workers. Many aspects of care are monitored using this approach. For example, we record temperatures, pulses and respiratory rate using graphs. We may also use this format to record aspects such as weight, fluid intake or hours of sleep.

We also use this information for comparison. For example, we may compare an increase in pulse rate with the temperature recording to identify if there are any identifiable trends. A rise in pulse rate noted may be associated with an increase in respiration or temperature. If this is not the case, other possible reasons for the

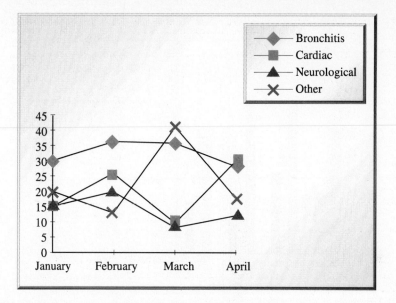

Figure 10.6 Graph to show hospital admissions from January to April.

increase in pulse rate may be considered. This normal, everyday, practice for health workers suggests that looking at graphs and analysing the observations noted is a common experience, an aspect that makes similar analysis in research terms relatively straightforward.

To help see how information can be translated into graph form it will be useful to review Figure 10.6. It can be seen that this graph indicates the number of admissions to the hospital ward in the months of January to April. Although this information is contained in Table 10.8 the graph has a stronger visual impact.

Histograms and bar graphs

These same data are presented in Figures 10.7 and 10.8 showing a histogram and a bar chart. *Histograms* offer an alternative means of presenting information for instant visual impact. Information is presented in a series of vertical columns adjacent to one another. *Bar charts* are similar to histograms except that the data presented in horizontal bars are presented separately with spaces between each measure.

In Figure 10.7, the example of a histogram, it can be noted that the horizontal axis has been used to record the time interval whilst the vertical axis has been used to note the frequency or number of observations made. It is accepted practice to present data in this way so that the frequency measure is along the vertical axis.

Also, it can be seen that the range of figures used in the vertical axis is a realistic representation of the number of observations made. In Figure 10.9 the number of years recorded is beyond the time of the study in the vertical column and large

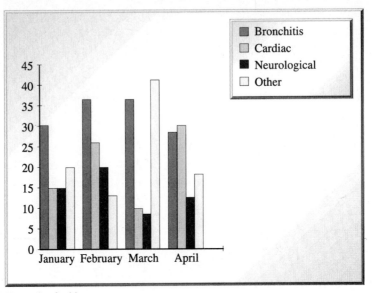

Figure 10.7 Example of a histogram.

numbers over and above the sample studied in the horizontal axis. This chart does
not support the information that is available, for the numbers are too small to be

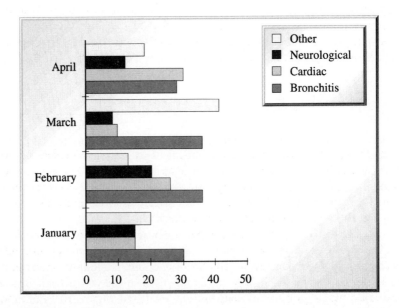

Figure 10.8 Example of a bar chart.

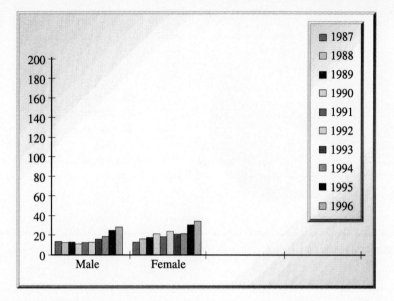

Figure 10.9 Poor graph design.

identified clearly in the numerical range given. This is an example of poor graph design which may seem to be a very obvious point and hardly worth noting in a book of this nature. However it has been included purposefully to introduce a word of caution into the text. Inexperienced researchers may not use graphs well when sharing their knowledge. It is important when reading research reports to examine the information supplied in both axes of a graph critically. It is very easy to show a line graph with very dramatic swings even when referring only to very small samples. Another important point to note is the importance of labelling graphs clearly when preparing research reports.

Pie charts

This is another popular way of presenting information for visual impact. As the name implies, presentation of information in this way can be likened to a pie. A circular picture is presented with slices to represent parts of the whole. An example of this format is noted in Figure 10.10 where the percentage of patient groups in a hospital ward (January to April, from Table 10.8) is indicated.

Although pie charts are a useful means of summarising information for visual impact it should be noted that it is not always easy to reflect data accurately in this approach, so it is perhaps used a little more cautiously by researchers than other methods of presentation.

There are other ways in which information may be visually presented following research projects but those outlined above reflect the most common. A good

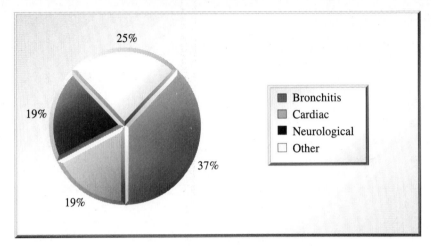

Figure 10.10 Example of a pie chart.

understanding of these basic principles will enhance the ability of those reading research reports to comprehend more complex patterns of presentation. The advent of computers in recent years has greatly enhanced the opportunities for researchers to explore the best way of presenting data visually in their own particular project. Computers will rapidly change the format of presentation from histograms and bar charts to pie charts and so on.

ACTIVITY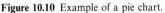

- Select a range of research articles that have used *qualitative* approaches to research and review how the data were collected and analysed.
- Is the interpretation clear?
- Select a range of research articles that have used *quantitative* approaches to research and presented data in statistical form.
- Look at the statistical results presented and consider whether they are presented in a clear, concise way.
- Is good use made of tables, graphs, etc.?

Summary

This chapter has given an overview of a range of approaches to data analysis in both qualitative and quantitative research. Additional information on this can be found in the further reading.

Further reading

Chenitz, W.C. and Swanson, J.M. (1986) *From Practice to Grounded Theory: Qualitative Research in Nursing*, Addison-Wesley, Menlo Park, California.

Clegg, F. (1987) *Simple Statistics. A Course Book for the Social Sciences*, Cambridge University Press, Cambridge.

Clifford, C. (1997) *Qualitative Research Methodology in Nursing and Health Care*, Open Learning Foundation/Churchill Livingstone, Edinburgh.

Clifford, C. and Harkin, L. (1997) *Inferential Statistics in Nursing and Health Care*, Open Learning Foundation/Churchill Livingstone, Edinburgh.

Dey, I. (1993) *Qualitative Data Analysis. A User-friendly Guide for Social Scientists*, Routledge, London.

Fielding, N.G. and Lee, R.M. (1991) *Using Computers in Qualitative Research*, Sage, London.

Field, P.A. and Morse, J. (1996) *Nursing Research: The Application of Qualitative Approaches*, Chapman & Hall, London.

Hicks, C. (1990) *Research and Statistics: A Practical Introduction for Nurses*, Prentice Hall, Hemel Hempstead.

Hinton, P.R. (1995) *Statistics Explained: A Guide for Social Science Students*, Routledge, London.

Keeble, S. (1995) *Experimental Research 1 and 2*, Open Learning Foundation/Churchill, Livingstone, Edinburgh.

Miles, M.B. and Hubermans, A.M. (1994) *Qualitative Data Analysis*, Sage, London.

Miller, H. (1995) *Descriptive Statistics*, Open Learning Foundation/Churchill Livingstone, Edinburgh.

Reid, N.G. and Boore, J.R.P. (1987) *Research Methods and Statistics in Health Care*, Edward Arnold, London.

Strauss, A. and Corbin, J. (1990) *Basics of Qualitative Research*, Sage, London.

Woodward, M. and Francis, L.M.A. (1988) *Statistics for Health Management and Research*, Edward Arnold, London.

11   Writing for research

In this chapter we will consider a range of issues relating to communicating research information. This may be seen as the final step in the research process and the first step in the process of dissemination and implementation which will be discussed further in the next chapter. We will discuss a number of issues relating to the following:

1. Writing for research.
2. Presenting research findings verbally to an audience.

When people undertake research for the first time they frequently experience more anxiety over the issues addressed in this chapter than any other part of their research studies. To help alleviate this anxiety the section on writing skills explores aspects of writing that may be demanded of health care practitioners undertaking research studies. Skills of presentation have been included because it is now fairly common for practitioners who have undertaken research studies to be asked to share their ideas, experiences or research results with their colleagues in a formal presentation.

Writing skills

Although it must be acknowledged that some people have more of a natural flair for writing than others, one reason why people might underestimate their ability to write well may simply be due to lack of practice. For many health care professionals approaching research studies for the first time it may have been some years since they were required to produce a formal piece of written work.

The purpose of writing is to convey ideas from one mind to another. If you wish to do this successfully and present written work in a way that is meaningful to the reader there are some guidelines that can help. These apply whether writing an essay, a research proposal, a research report or an article for publication.

Essay writing

It is quite a common practice for students undertaking research studies to be asked to produce an essay for their first piece of assessed work. The purpose of this is twofold. In the first instance it allows the student to begin to practise the writing skills required for the course. Secondly, it allows the teacher to assess the student's ability to write at the academic level required on the particular course of study whilst also assessing the individual student's level of understanding of the given topic. Because of this approach in research courses some general guidelines for essay writing are outlined below.

Planning

The planning stage is crucial in the writing process and yet it is one that is often neglected. Quite commonly, in poor essays, the writer has no obvious systematic plan and the overall structure of the piece of work is poor. If the writer changes from one subject to another in an erratic fashion, the reader may be unable to understand the ideas presented in the essay.

The writer may be clear in his or her own mind as to what he or she wants to say yet be failing to do this in a way in which the reader can understand. When planning an essay it is useful to follow some very simple guidelines.

Be sure that the topic of the essay is clearly understood

It is easy to get side-tracked when writing essays and if this happens the writer may fail to address the title of the essay. It is useful to highlight relevant points in the title or question by underlining them. As work is being prepared it is useful to keep asking whether key issues are being addressed.

Read any relevant literature pertaining to the subject

When reading, take notes, or underline, any relevant factors that could be included in the essay. The amount and nature of the literature read at this stage will depend on the academic requirements of the course. If you were undertaking a master's degree programme for example, the expectation will be higher than if you were doing an essay as part of a short course of study into the research process (we will return to this below).

Write a plan

Following the review of the literature think about the topic in detail and consider all relevant aspects that may be discussed. At this stage make notes of the order of priority that will be given to the points raised.

Review the plan

Review the plan and consider whether there are clearly defined sections and if the sequence of information is logical.

Write a draft essay

This is a very important stage when essay writing. The student who is able to produce a perfect piece of work at first attempt is a very rare breed indeed. Although some of us may aspire to such ability it is far more common for good pieces of written work to have gone through several revisions before the writer feels that he or she has fully completed the work.

An increasing number of people now have access to word processors. These can be a very valuable tool when writing and editing work and can, in the long term, save a lot of energy when reviewing draft documents.

A useful tip at this stage is to write the essay on one side of paper only. This will allow the order, or structure, of the essay to be changed if, on revision, it is felt that the work does not flow logically from topic to topic. The 'cut and paste' orders in word processing packs allow you to do this very simply if you are writing on a computer. Otherwise, if you are restricted to hand-written pages the order can be simply changed by cutting out the relevant sections of the essay, and transferring them to a more appropriate spot (i.e. cutting and pasting!).

Another tip is to leave plenty of space between the lines of writing. Use the double spacing facility if you have access to a computer or use alternate lines if handwriting on lined paper. This will enable corrections to be made in such a way that work can be read when the amendments are done.

There are several advantages of writing a draft copy. The first is that the writer will be able to scrutinise the work critically to see if the plan has been followed and that the meaning is clear. Secondly, in writing a draft copy, the writer has some information at hand to share with a supervisor or teacher who will be able to give advice on how to progress. If a teacher is not available there may be a colleague who is prepared to give peer support and constructively comment on a draft essay. Alternatively, it is useful to pace writing in such a way that once the draft copy has been completed, it can be put to one side for a few days. The writer can then return to the work and review it. It is frequently the case that a break from written work helps the writer approach it from a fresh perspective and see it more from a 'reader's eye'. When reviewing a draft copy the following points should be considered.

1. The introduction should be clearly related to the essay title and clarify any issues within that. Any ideas or concepts that will be used in the essay should be stated and some indication given as to the depth in which issues will be explored in the essay. This can be done in a brief overview of the content of the essay.
2. The structure of the essay should then be analysed. It should be noted first whether the essay progresses logically and systematically. If this is so then each paragraph will be written around a theme or sub-theme. Sentences should be simple and related to one idea only. Arguments for and against points made should be clearly stated and appropriate evidence given to support points made. An academic essay should not be a collection of unsupported opinions; it should be a well-reasoned and balanced discussion in which issues are discussed in an objective and critical manner.

3. The use of literature in the text should be appropriate and the writer should clearly note when information has been used from other sources. Failure to do this may be interpreted as plagiarism. Some of key points relevant to referencing information in an essay are outlined below.

    (a) If a direct quote is used from another source, indent the lines used or use quotation marks. It can be seen in printed texts that when this is done, the line spacing and/or letter size is altered to ensure the quotation stands out clearly from the main body of the text:

    'This quote has been directly copied from a book on the art of nursing research and consequently has been presented in this format on this page'

    (b) If ideas from another source are used, but not the exact words of the original author, the information, or ideas, can be incorporated into the writing and credit to the source material at end of the account.

    It was suggested earlier that you seek additional information about referencing from your local library. In summary writers may choose to make references by indicating the name of the author and the date of publication at the end of the section, e.g. (Bloggs 1989). This is known as the Harvard system. Alternatively they may choose to use the numerical approach, or Vancouver system, of indicating references in which names and dates are not necessarily included in the text but listed by number like this[1] and listed numerically at the end of the paper in the reference list.

4. The writing style is important when writing for academic purposes. Essays written for academic purposes are generally written in the third person. One of the difficulties when writing in the first person is that it personalises work in such a way that it is not evident to the reader that the writer is presenting information objectively. If the writer were to say 'I think research is ...' it does not indicate that others may also have identified similar trends. Statements such as 'It has been suggested that research is ...' or 'there is evidence to suggest that research is ...' can be used to overcome this and to present written work in a more objective fashion.

    The writer should take care to ensure that a consistent approach is used throughout the essay.

5. When writing essays the use of complicated jargon should be avoided. A good guide is never to use a complicated word, or number of words, when a simple one will make the point just as well. This word of caution is particularly important for prospective researchers as one of the reasons given in Chapter 2 for failure to spread research findings is that the language used may be too complex for many practitioners to understand. Although there are occasions when it is difficult to avoid technical language, the writing should always be presented in a way that is meaningful to the audience it is being prepared for.

6. The conclusion of an essay should be unambiguous and relate clearly to the content of the essay. The writer should refer back to the points made in the introduction, summarise what has been said about these in the discussion and base the final conclusion on the evidence that has been presented in the essay.

7. A full reference list should accompany the essay. The purpose of this, as noted above, is to give credit to any other work incorporated into the essay. In addition the reference list gives a source of information to the reader wishing to explore ideas highlighted in the work.

Completing the essay

Only when a thorough editorial review, or critique, of the draft essay has been done is the student ready to write the final piece of work. All of the points noted above should have been considered. The end result, the completed essay, should be a neat, logical and well-balanced piece of work.

Writing for research

If you have mastered the skills required for writing a good academic essay then you will be easily able to transfer that knowledge to writing for research. Specific areas that will be explored in this section are writing a research proposal and writing a research report. Before we explore these, however, it is worth briefly outlining what is expected in a literature review for this is crucial to any writing for research.

Literature review/critique

The purpose of completing a literature review and critique was outlined in Chapter 6. At the outset it is helpful to consider the distinction between a literature review and a literature critique. The former is simply that – an overview of the literature available whilst a critique will be more focused on the research methodologies adopted in the literature and the 'quality' of the research reported. A critique will enable you to demonstrate your knowledge of research in answering the question of whether the research design is appropriate for the question asked and whether this has been considered from an appropriate theoretical base.

In a research critique it is common for the researcher to go through the piece of research in a step-by-step way, examining each component to the research design.

An important point to remember is that a research critique is just that – a critical review of the research, not a criticism of the researcher who has written the report. Moreover, the use of critical reviews as a method of teaching about research can sometimes leave students with the feeling that very little research will stand up to critical scrutiny. However, it is important to look for strengths as well as weaknesses in overall research design. It is also important to remember that it would be very rare for one piece of research to have a major impact on practice – it is the collective findings of several pieces of work that will do that if appropriate. It might be helpful for you to note that the term used by researchers involved in a large-scale critiquing exercise of research reports is *meta-analysis.* In this situation the researcher combines the results from several studies to determine the collective findings.

Why review the literature?

A literature review may be undertaken for a variety of reasons. For example, it may be undertaken to identify the range of past research studies and to summarise the present state of knowledge, to differentiate between commentary and research, or to identify the theoretical base of research. Reading the literature on a topic will help the intending researcher avoid rediscovering the wheel and making the same mistakes. It may help the researcher to get new insights into new methods that may be used to study the topic and, finally, from this perspective it may help focus research questions.

   At a practical level the findings from the research literature can be used to influence practice or, in the absence of sufficient research, recommend further research. They may also be used to support the rationale for undertaking or replicating a research study. In addition it is common practice for students learning about research to be asked to undertake a literature search and to write a review of this as part of their course work.

When to do a literature review

The question of when to do a literature review will yield a range of responses depending firstly on the orientation of the research. Some approaches to qualitative research do not recommend that a review is completed until some of the data relating to the topic of study are collected. However, for the quantitatively orientated researcher the approach is somewhat different. In this case the researcher will complete a review at the beginning; for most it is necessary that the review is ongoing throughout a study. This is particularly important in research projects that are extending over a period of time as the state of knowledge can develop rapidly during the course of a study. Finally, for the same reason it is important to undertake a literature review at the end of a study.

How to do a literature review

The first thing to clarify when writing a literature review as part of a course work assignment is to determine the required length of the work and the expected completion date. If a thousand-word assignment has to be produced in a four week period then the detail in the work will not be comparable to a literature search incorporated in a Ph.D. thesis. This may seem to be a very obvious statement, but all too often students undertaking a literature search for the first time get very involved with the subject and gather so much information that it is impossible to utilise this adequately in a written review. The skills of synthesising knowledge can be developed with practice. It is not true that the more references available in a piece of work the better it is. Sometimes the reverse is true, for too much information may only serve to confuse. What is important is that relevant information is used well. Quality not quantity is a good guide when preparing a literature review.

The literature review should have an introduction, a discussion section and a conclusion. The introduction should inform the reader of the subject area, how the literature search was undertaken and what sources of information were utilised in this, for example, that a computer search was instigated. The skills required to search literature were discussed briefly in Chapter 6. Once you start to collect material to review you will begin to identify 'leads' in the papers or books you are reading that will help direct your reading. It is important to follow up leads but avoid 'overkill'; in other words, to know when to stop. Another thing to look out for is the seminal sources of material in the references: the key references or theories that have influenced your subject area. It will also help in your review of the literature if you keep focusing on the key questions you are addressing in order to narrow your search.

The volume of research material in some subject areas is enormous and writers will need to clarify in the introduction exactly what constraints they have faced and what measures have been taken to overcome these. For example, the volume of research work undertaken into pressure area care is very large, consequently a review of literature in this area may be very specific, focusing perhaps on one particular treatment. Again this is where advice from a supervisor is helpful. It has been suggested several times, for example, that time available may place constraints on developing a study. Linked to this is the nature of the research. For example if doing a major research study at M.Phil. or Ph.D. level it would be expected that all relevant sources of literature be examined in a review. In contrast the student on an undergraduate programme may have major limitations in terms of time to do a study and so may need to set parameters on the time spent on searching the literature. Consequently, in smaller-scale studies it is not unusual for researchers to indicate that the range of literature used was limited to a specific time span or locality.

The literature review should clearly relate to the area of research interest. Previously published research on the subject should be summarised and analysed. When reading a wide range of literature on a topic it is commonly found that specific views, or themes, can be identified. As such themes emerge, it is useful to group studies together as this tends to provide a structure for the written work. All views should be represented in an unbiased literature review. Both sides of an argument, or conflicting research results, should be presented, even if they conflict with the writer's own beliefs on a subject.

The conclusion to a literature review can be short but should, as in essay writing, summarise the key points. The difference, however, in a literature review is the conclusion will commonly point out any deficits in the literature and lead to perhaps an identified need for any deficits to be addressed by research in the future.

A full and accurate *reference list* should be available at the end of the literature review. Many new research students ask how many references should be used. The answer to this is usually ambiguous as it really does depend on a number of things, not least the subject area. For example, if a researcher is exploring an area that has not previously been the subject of a research study it is unlikely that he or she will be able to identify many references. In contrast if a researcher is approaching a topic that has been well researched he or she might find the range of references is very wide. Experience would indicate that research projects undertaken as part of an undergraduate programme of study may need in the range of 20–100 references, whilst at the other end of the spectrum, projects at M.Phil. or Ph.D. level can range between 50 and 500. The important point to remember here is that the number of references depends on the available literature. If there is limited research literature available on a given topic this would serve to support the need to build up a body of literature through research. In this case the literature review will focus on commentary articles, but here you need to make the distinction between such articles and research. If appropriate related literature may be used to illustrate a point. Linked with this, an important point to remember is that quality, not quantity, is usually the key to a good literature review.

Research proposal

It is normal practice to write a research proposal prior to undertaking a research study. Broadly speaking there are several reasons why nursing and health workers may be required to do this:

1. As part of an assessed course of study of research methods.
2. As an application for funds to support the development of the research project.
3. When seeking permission from an ethical committee to undertake a study in a clinical setting.

Even if there is no formal demand on the researcher to write a proposal prior to the study it is still a useful exercise for it helps to focus on the key issues in the research and facilitates the planning of the study in providing a structured outline of intent.

Generally speaking, however, the way in which you might prepare a proposal for all these purposes varies with a different emphasis on each section of the proposal. For example, if health care students are undertaking a course of study in which the focus is on learning about research design, the assessment of learning may be very broad in scope, focusing on the students' ability to read the literature critically and to understand the broad principles of planning a research study. Consequently there may be great emphasis on the literature review within the proposal, with perhaps two-thirds of the proposal concentrating on related literature and leading into a justification of the research. In contrast, if applying for funds for research the funding body usually has a very prescribed pattern of presenting the proposal: it may only allow a very short discussion of related literature and place greater emphasis on the overall research design and feasibility of the study.

Before preparing a research proposal it is important that the requirements of the 'audience' it is being written for are clarified as the approach may differ slightly. Many organisations offering grants for research purposes have their own format for research proposals and will include this in the information pack sent to applicants. The same is true of ethical committees. It is in the researcher's own interest to follow the preferred style of the group to which he or she is presenting the research proposal.

Failure to do so when seeking funding support will almost certainly result in the proposal being rejected at the outset. Failure to do so for an ethical committee is likely to result in the proposal being returned with a polite request to complete it on the correct forms. This would of course result in delay in processing the proposal through the committee which in turn will result in a delay to develop the research.

Preparing a research proposal

Whatever the purpose of writing the research proposal there are some key points to remember if you wish to develop your skill in this area. This obviously includes a clear vision of the purpose and process involved in the proposed research. However, many potential researchers have the vision but lack the skill required to present this to those people who may be reading the proposed study. Consequently an important skill in presenting a proposal is the ability to write in a concise, logical manner avoiding the use of jargon. Remember that use of jargon will not help the application if the committee approving the proposals have difficulty in understanding the subject. Indeed many of the guidelines sent by funding bodies to prospective researchers now specify that any proposal submitted should be written in a style that would be understood by non-professional members of any committee as such members participate in the decision-making process, deciding whether or not to support the proposal through a funding committee or an ethics committee.

Linked with this is the overall style of presentation. Although ultimately it is true that any judgement on a proposed research study will be made on the quality of the overall research plan, the style of presentation will enhance your chances of getting to the point at which your proposal is considered. Again it may be a simple matter of following the guidelines set; for example if you are asked to present a proposal that is typed but instead you choose to present a hand-written proposal you will not be doing yourself a service. Also it is worth remembering that the computers and word processing packages now available in many homes have resulted in an increased expectation in terms of the typed work that is produced. You can test this for yourself if you can find some papers that were typed and printed on one of the early word processing packages and compare them with the quality that is available today.

In terms of the three reasons for completing research proposals above we have already discussed the ethical issues in Chapter 4. If you are completing a research proposal for a piece of assessed work on a programme of studies we will assume that you have already got access to a supervisor or lecturer who will specify guidelines as to the expectation for the project. Consequently we are left with writing a proposal to secure funds to support a research project and it is worth briefly considering the key features that will be considered in such a proposal:

1. The overall worth of the proposed project.
2. The overall research design.
3. Project management – the ability of the researcher to complete the project proposed.

Proposals will be sent to external assessors to review. These assessors will be very skilled at reviewing research proposals and in addition will have a particular expertise in the area of the research or in the proposed research methodology.

The first point to make in terms of the overall worth of a given project is that the emphasis placed on this will vary according to the source of funding. For example, it may be that the funds are available to support a specific project that has been developed by the funding body – in this case they will have already decided on the overall worth of the project in offering it out for tender (invited bids for a researcher to complete the work). Examples of both these kinds of funding can be found in most sources of funds in the United Kingdom (see Chapter 4). For example, the NHS R&D strategy has created opportunities for researchers to submit to a wide range of subject areas at national and local level. Judgement on the overall worth of the proposed project relates to identified priority areas for the funding body. There would be little value in submitting proposals that fell outside clearly stated priorities. As an extreme example, a funding body supporting research into people who had a physical disability would have little interest in proposals exploring aspects of mental disability.

The overall research design relates to the overall standard of the research proposed which we will discuss in a little more detail below. An external assessor would be interested in whether it is a coherent plan, consistent in presentation, and realistic in the time frames proposed. They would of course focus specifically on the research design to determine whether it is a reliable and valid method of approaching the area of study.

The final section, the project management, relates to two aspects. First is whether the funding allocated for the project is appropriately distributed. Secondly, the management potential of the applicant/s will be assessed, possibly at two levels. The first is the ability of the researcher to undertake the project. Decisions regarding this are made on the basis of past experience – a track record in the field of study. The second, which is more applicable for the newcomer to research, relates to the individual potential of the researcher in terms of developing research expertise. This links to the support available to the researcher in terms of supervision. Thus, if as a newcomer to research you were submitting a proposal for funding for a project you want to develop you will be judged on your merit but also the person or team who is supervising you will also be judged to determine if the appropriate support to develop your potential will be provided.

In general terms the research proposal follows the stages of the research process and so there are similarities with a research report. The research proposal is, however, written in the future tense whilst the research report would be written in the past tense.

Guidelines outlining the presentation of a research proposal are summarised in Figure 11.1.

The *title* of the research proposal study should clearly reflect the subject of the study. It is quite tempting to spend time thinking up good literary titles for proposed research studies but these do little to focus the reader or to provide a clear indication of the focus of the study for future indexing of the research in library services. For example the title 'Bad experience' may catch the eye in a shelf of fictional books but it will not tell future researchers that the contents reflect a study of communication

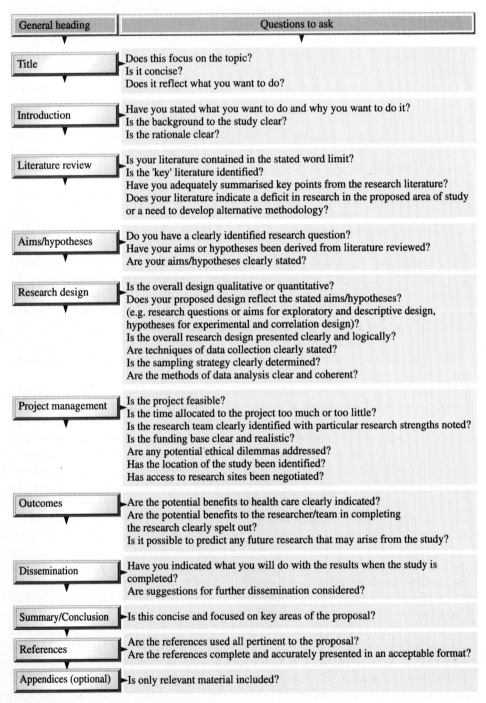

General heading	Questions to ask
Title	Does this focus on the topic? Is it concise? Does it reflect what you want to do?
Introduction	Have you stated what you want to do and why you want to do it? Is the background to the study clear? Is the rationale clear?
Literature review	Is your literature contained in the stated word limit? Is the 'key' literature identified? Have you adequately summarised key points from the research literature? Does your literature indicate a deficit in research in the proposed area of study or a need to develop alternative methodology?
Aims/hypotheses	Do you have a clearly identified research question? Have your aims or hypotheses been derived from literature reviewed? Are your aims/hypotheses clearly stated?
Research design	Is the overall design qualitative or quantitative? Does your proposed design reflect the stated aims/hypotheses? (e.g. research questions or aims for exploratory and descriptive design, hypotheses for experimental and correlation design)? Is the overall research design presented clearly and logically? Are techniques of data collection clearly stated? Is the sampling strategy clearly determined? Are the methods of data analysis clear and coherent?
Project management	Is the project feasible? Is the time allocated to the project too much or too little? Is the research team clearly identified with particular research strengths noted? Is the funding base clear and realistic? Are any potential ethical dilemmas addressed? Has the location of the study been identified? Has access to research sites been negotiated?
Outcomes	Are the potential benefits to health care clearly indicated? Are the potential benefits to the researcher/team in completing the research clearly spelt out? Is it possible to predict any future research that may arise from the study?
Dissemination	Have you indicated what you will do with the results when the study is completed? Are suggestions for further dissemination considered?
Summary/Conclusion	Is this concise and focused on key areas of the proposal?
References	Are the references used all pertinent to the proposal? Are the references complete and accurately presented in an acceptable format?
Appendices (optional)	Is only relevant material included?

Figure 11.1 Planning a research proposal: key areas for consideration.

in hospital settings. You need to ensure the title reflects what you are going to do. So in our example here a more appropriate title might be 'Communication in an acute hospital'. The title should also be as concise as possible. You will realise the value of this if you do proceed with a study – the longer the title the more frustrating it becomes when you move on to tell other people about the project, not to mention the hours spent typing it out when preparing reports.

The *introduction* to the research proposal should clearly state what you want to do and why. The background to the proposed study should be stated indicating why there is a need for this particular work to be done. This will set the proposed study into a suitable context for discussion. The rationale for undertaking a study at this moment in time should also be considered as this serves as a justification for the research. So, for example, if you want to do a study that meets a regional needs for health care research in an area where there is a deficit of research completed, the background would indicate this and the rationale would arise out of this as a justification for the research to be done.

The *literature review* is the next step. The purpose of completing a literature review is to find out what work has been done before, to find out if there are any 'gaps' in the literature and to review the research methods that may have been adopted to research into the area of interest. Completion of a literature review when preparing a research report will indicate whether there are any gaps in the research in the area or whether there are any gaps in the research methods that have been adopted. For example, research into one aspect of health care may have included qualitative studies but little in the way of quantifiable data or vice versa.

Although it may not be demanded as a separate section in all research proposals, a review of the literature serves to support the rationale for undertaking the research. The first thing you need to check here is the length of the literature review. For example, if you are completing a research proposal as a piece of assessed course work then you may be expected to include a long literature review in this, for example, 2000–3000 words. In contrast if you are responding to a request for research proposal to a funding body for research the literature review may be kept very brief, simply outlining some of the key work related to the subject area and the relevance of this to the proposed study. The important point in developing the literature review is to ensure that the most important research literature pertaining to your topic is included – take care to distinguish between commentaries and research.

The *aims* or *hypotheses* for the proposed study will be derived from any deficits noted in the literature and the rationale for completing the study in the first instance. Remember that you will use a hypothesis for experimental or correlational design whilst you might state aims or research questions for descriptive designs.

The next area to consider is the proposed *research design*. By this point the reader of your proposal will be looking for consistency in approach and will be interested to see whether your stated aims or hypotheses can be addressed in the research design proposed. For example, if a hypothesis was proposed that a new method of rehabilitation would enhance the recovery rate of people with head injuries but then went on to describe a research design that was largely qualitative in orientation and focusing on feelings rather than outcomes, the reader might assume a limited insight into the research design.

The techniques of data collection should be clearly spelt out. As indicated in Chapter 9, in health care this may include use of questionnaires, interviews, observation or reviews of records. If using a range of techniques it is important to indicate why a mixed approach has been chosen and how each part will fit into the total purpose of the study.

The population should be identified and the sampling strategies that will be adopted clearly stated. As indicated in Chapters 6, 8 and 9 this can be variable depending on the overall research design. This will have an impact on the proposed method of analysing data which should be noted.

The next section will involve issues related to *project management*. This refers to the overall organisational issues that may impact on developing the project. This includes general questions relating to the feasibility of the project; for example, whether the time allocated to the completion of the project is sufficient and whether the researcher or research team have the skills to complete the project. Project management includes consideration of how funds will be managed (see Chapter 4).

Within the project management section any anticipated ethical dilemmas should be noted, as should any action taken to overcome them (see Chapter 4). In addition to this, access to research sites should be outlined. It is important that the distinction between ethical issues and issues relating to access are clarified. Even if you have got approval of a research ethics committee to proceed with your research this does not mean you have access – this has to be negotiated through managerial channels. For example, if you wanted to study aspects of health care in the community you might have got permission to approach patients from an ethical point of view but before you can do so you will still need permission of the management team in the community unit.

Depending on the overall research design the potential or expected *outcomes* of the research results should be noted. These can be a challenge to identify but there is an increasing emphasis in research projects for a researcher to indicate them. This is because a clear statement of potential outcomes for the researcher serves to indicate whether the costs involved in supporting a project is indicative of money that would be well spent.

The final area for consideration is that of *dissemination*, how you are going to help the process of ensuring that people will hear about your research. We will consider this further in Chapter 12.

As with all other pieces of written work it may be appropriate to write a brief *summary* or *conclusion*. This could be used to emphasise important points and reinforce the perceived value in undertaking the study proposed.

Finally there is the potential for using *appendices* when preparing a research proposal, but again before doing so check the guidelines that are available to you. Some funding bodies are very strict about the length of the proposal including all material whilst others may be more flexible. If appendices are used in research proposals it is generally for such things as the *curriculum vitae* of the researcher or the research team. This is used to support the case that proposes that the team has the relevant experience to manage the project proposed.

Another way in which appendices may be used is to include any draft instruments such as questionnaires that may be used to support the proposal and any information relating to information sheets for the sample group (see Chapter 4).

Research report

The pattern adopted to write a research report reflects that used to write a research proposal (see Figure 11.2). The report is written in the past tense and, obviously, contains more detail than a research proposal as all aspects of the research process will be discussed. In the section on research proposals three sections were identified: an introduction, in which the aims or hypothesis are clearly stated and the background to the study explained; a review of the literature; and a section on proposed methodology.

When writing the research report the researcher would elaborate on all of these sections. The *results* of the study will be presented. The volume of data included in this section is left to the discretion of the researcher. Although it may be seen as ideal to exhibit all of the data gathered during the course of a research study, this may cause the text to become very complex. To overcome this, researchers frequently use tables and graphs as these offer a shorthand way of presenting data. An alternative approach is to summarise findings and include the results in appendices at the end of the research report so that data are available for reference purposes.

If the researcher has stated a hypothesis, he or she may state in the section giving the research results whether it has been accepted or rejected. Otherwise the presentation of results includes an interpretation of findings initially. The advantage of this to readers of research reports is that they can read this section objectively to determine what they feel to be the outcome of the research.

The final section in a research report is the *discussion*. At this point the researcher discusses the results obtained in the context of the aims of the research, the research setting and in relation to any other background information highlighted in the literature review. Aspects related to the research methodology can be highlighted with specific emphasis being placed on any particularly interesting results.

Within the final discussion the researcher should acknowledge any limitations to the study that may have affected the final outcome. Throughout the study note should be taken of ensuring anonymity and confidentiality of the people participating in the research.

Finally the researcher will consider any recommendations he or she wishes to make as a result of the study. This may, for example, be a recommendation specifically related to the subject of the research, or alternatively, to research design in future studies.

Many research studies leave the researcher with more questions than answers and it is not uncommon for the closing lines of a research report to indicate a need for further study into an area of practice.

At the end of a research report a complete and accurate list of *references* should be included.

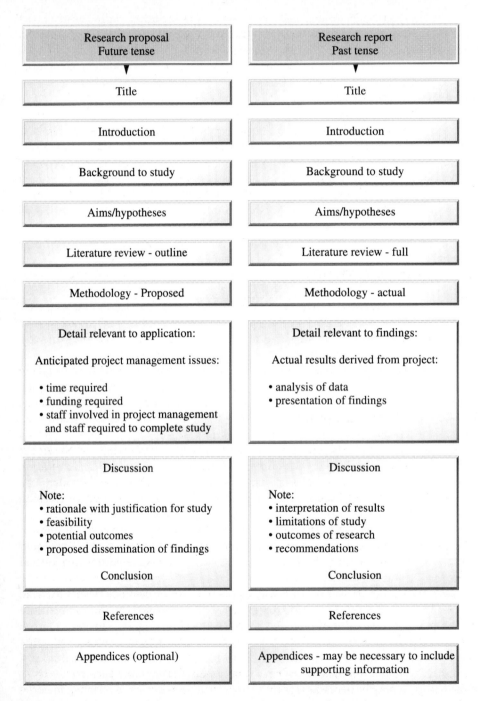

Figure 11.2 A comparison between a research proposal and a research report.

If the researcher has used material to create an *appendix* this would complete the report and be included after the reference section. The appendices are generally used to hold any information seen as relevant to the study as a whole but not so essential that they should be incorporated in the main text. For example, letters asking for permission to undertake a study are not necessarily included in the text of a report but are important to refer to when describing the overall research design. Also, as noted above, it may be distracting to put all the research data into a report, yet this may need to be available for reference purposes.

The information outlined above provides a general guideline for writing research reports. Examination of many published research texts will reveal that although the format noted above will be identifiable in some reports, others will have a different structure. Ultimately the researcher will plan the specific format of the report based on the structure of the research study overall.

Writing for publication

All people who undertake research studies do need to consider how to share their findings with their colleagues. One very obvious way to reach a wide audience is to prepare a research report for publication. The following information is given as a guideline for those who may wish to publish their research work.

The first thing to decide is which journal to submit a paper to, as this helps clarify the audience for which the article is being written. If this is not done a paper may need to be rewritten to meet the needs of the target audience of a particular journal. All journals produce their own guidelines for contributors. In many journals these are included on the back page of each copy whilst for others there may be a need to write to the editor for this information. The journal guidelines advise on the length of the article, the writing style, the preferred referencing system and the presentation of tables and graphs. It is normal practice for journals to request at least two manuscripts which have been typed in double spacing. This is to facilitate editorial work.

It may be worth contacting the editor before writing an article to determine whether there would be sufficient interest to publish the paper. If the researcher has explored a very specialist subject area, for example, it may not be seen as relevant to a journal with a very general readership. Alternatively if the editor feels that a particular topic has received sufficient coverage in recent months he or she may not be interested in publishing another report on the topic at this moment in time. If this is known at the outset it can save a lot of time and energy for both the writer and the reviewer.

When writing for publication the guidelines given in the previous section still apply and a similar format followed. If writing a research report for publication, however, the researcher would need to consider the emphasis that is placed on each section of the report. It may be necessary for them to determine priorities in selecting material for inclusion in the article and the weighting given to each section may need to be adjusted to match the word limit of the finished article. The length of journal articles varies but 2000–3000 words is a fairly average length for publication.

In any article submitted for publication, particular note should be taken of anonymity. In offering confidentiality to research subjects when undertaking studies the researcher should ensure that this is not breached by a slip of the pen in preparing an article. It is a useful exercise to read some research reports in journals to see how confidentiality is maintained in these. In so doing a pattern can be identified in which such terms as 'A Health Centre in the Midlands' or 'A group of nurses in a large teaching hospital' are used to give anonymity whilst also setting into context the location of the study.

The researcher would be expected to write an abstract to accompany the article. This is a short summary of the project and should give a very succinct overview in approximately 150 words. In this the purpose and results of the study should be made clear to the reader. The value of an abstract is that it allows the reader to determine whether the contents of a paper are relevant to them. Some journals ask authors to identify key words that will both focus the reader and help when indexing the article.

It is also a matter of courtesy for the writer to consider any support, help or co-operation that has been received during the course of the study. This may have been from research subjects, a supervisor or from a source of funding given to the study. It is accepted practice to acknowledge such support given at the end of an article.

When articles are submitted for publication the writers are advised to keep a copy. This is essential in the first instance because papers can get lost in transit and, if that were to happen without another copy being retained, all the hard work involved in preparation will be wasted. A second good reason for keeping a copy is that when an article is published it is useful to review how much editorial work has been done on it. This will help the writer to gauge his or her own skills in writing for this medium and may therefore be a useful learning experience. You are not advised to submit work to more than one journal at a time as this can lead to complications in the area of copyright if the work is accepted for publication by more than one journal.

Once an article has been submitted for publication the writer should be prepared for a long wait before final confirmation of acceptance or rejection. Most journals operate a system of review in which articles are sent out to a professional panel which determines suitability for publication. This system does have positive benefits but it is quite a time-consuming process. If the journal does accept an article it may do so provisionally, dependent on some modification or it may accept it as it is. Once it is accepted the writer is asked to sign a contract which clarifies issues related to publication and copyright of the material when published.

Publishing material is not an easy process for there is a lot of demand on a limited amount of space. Consequently researchers need to consider other ways in which information can be shared. As this includes presenting information verbally, the next section concentrates on presentation skills.

Presentation skills

This section has been included in this book on research because of the responsibility held by the researcher to ensure that research findings are shared with as wide an audience as possible. Before exploring this topic it is worth stressing that anybody interested in undertaking some research of their own must anticipate that there will come a time when they will be expected to share their findings in a lecture format, be that in a classroom as a lecture or seminar, or in a conference.

The skills of verbal presentation can be developed with practice. It is hoped that the information included in this section will help newcomers to research to develop the skills required to share their knowledge with others in a meaningful way. It is not unusual for anyone asked to speak publicly for the first time to experience extreme anxiety. However, following the first experience most will admit they have gained a lot of confidence. A little anxiety before public speaking is seen by some to be important, for this can be constructive and helps to motivate the speaker towards a more polished performance. If the speaker does not feel some anxiety they may demonstrate an over-confident approach that can lead to a poor presentation.

There is no doubt that public speaking is a nerve racking experience but anxieties related to this can be markedly reduced if the speaker is well prepared and so the following sections give guidelines on the skills required to give a good presentation.

Preparing a lecture

The principles of presenting information apply regardless of the subject matter, be that a research report or a lecture on a more general subject area. For convenience the term 'lecture' is used in this section to illustrate the points made in relation to presenting information to a group. Where appropriate information specific to the presentation of research papers will be given.

Organisational factors

1. The first step in preparation is to *clarify the topic* of the lecture. It is important to make sure that the speaker and the organiser have the same expectation of the content of the talk. If a timetable for the day is available this can be consulted to ensure that there is no overlap with the subject area and the presentation of any other speaker. If there are areas of similarity it is important that these are discussed at an early stage in preparation so that any repetition of subject material is avoided.
2. Clarify how much *time* is allocated for the presentation. Lecture time allocated can vary. An hour is a fairly common time period for many situations to which researchers are invited to share their findings with small groups. However, only fifteen minutes may be allocated to present a research paper at a conference and it is obviously crucial that this is known beforehand. In conferences that are tightly scheduled it is normal for the chairman to stop the speaker when the allocated time is used. If the speaker was not fully prepared for this he or she might not have got beyond the introduction! It is even harder for a speaker to be prepared for fifteen minutes and find that the organisers expect the session to last an hour!

3. Make sure the audience *mix* is known. This allows the speaker to adjust the presentation to match the level of knowledge of the audience. It may be assumed, for example, that there is a different level of knowledge in a group of trained staff compared with a group of students who have just started their course of training. If the level of presentation is inappropriate then the audience can become restless and this can be very distracting for the speaker.
4. Identify the *venue* of the lecture. This is probably best done nearer the time of the lecture but is included here as a relevant organisational factor. If it is possible, identifying the venue of the lecture may give opportunity to explore the facilities available before speaking. It is useful to check the acoustics in the room if possible. If it is a large area it may be useful for the speaker to take a friend or colleague to sit on a back row to see if the presentation can be heard in a full rehearsal. There may be a need to practice voice projection for example. Alternatively, if there is a microphone available it might be helpful to practise using this so that it is a familiar tool by the time the lecture commences.

    If travelling some distance to give a lecture some of these points may have to be checked on the day. However it is important to check travel arrangements and parking facilities if appropriate as a last minute rush can cause added anxiety.

Preparing the lecture paper

Having clarified the organisational aspects the researcher can concentrate on preparing the paper for presentation. The principles of public speaking are the same as those of writing. When preparing a paper for a lecture the introduction should *set the scene*; the main body of the talk should *discuss key issues*; the conclusion should *summarise* what has been said.

If giving an outline of a research project the researcher will need to determine priorities, for if allocated a short time there may not be sufficient time to cover all aspects of a study. A source of reference for an audience can do much to reduce the frustrations that occur as a result of time limitation for a presentation. For example it may be possible to refer the audience to the original research report which may be available to them, even if in an unpublished format.

When preparing material for a lecture it is fairly common for the first draft to have too much detail included. This is not a bad thing for it serves to ensure that the knowledge base of the speaker is quite wide. This helps the individual level of confidence, particularly when questions are invited from an audience.

Following critical review of the draft content the lecture should be adjusted to match the time available. The key headings should be clearly identified and then the method of presentation considered.

Method of presentation

Speakers are generally invited to talk on a topic that reflects an area of special interest to them. This makes both preparation and presentation easier, for interest tends to inspire enthusiasm. It is important, however, to be wary of an over-enthusiastic approach for this, too, can be detrimental to a presentation!

The key factor in considering how to present a lecture is to think of ways in which the interest of the audience can be retained. It is useful for anybody involved in presenting information to note the strengths and weaknesses of any lecture sessions that they have attended. This usually gives clues as to what may be considered good techniques to adopt. The points noted below are not exhaustive by any means but contain some useful tips for the newcomer to public speaking:

1. It is not generally advisable to read the paper, word for word, to an audience. On occasion this approach works quite well, but frequently the result is a presentation which does little to capture the imagination of the audience. A compromise can be reached by identifying key headings from a written paper and using these to guide the presentation. If this is done the result is likely to be a more relaxed approach (as long as the presenter does not try to memorise word for word what is written on the paper!). Audio-visual aids can be used to help remember detail and to explain more complex issues such as research results. The use of these will be discussed in more detail later.

2. Rehearse a presentation beforehand. The use of a tape recorder helps with this for it is possible to check back and critically review the content of the lecture. Of course it is never quite the same rehearsing in the privacy of the home environment as in front of an audience, but this rehearsal can certainly help exclude those words or awkward phrases that are likely to cause problems when public speaking. In addition it might inspire the speaker to change the tone of voice if the presentation sounds monotonous on tape. Also the timing of a presentation can be adjusted as this type of rehearsal allows speakers to check on how long their presentations last.

3. Avoid jargon. When presenting information the same advice on the use of jargon as that given in the section on writing skills applies. Do not use complex words when simple ones will do. The use of jargon can serve to alienate the speaker from the audience. If presenting a research paper it is important to remember that what might be everyday language to a researcher will not necessarily be so to an audience.

4. Body language is another important point to consider, for this tends to give the audience a lot of clues about the individual presenting the paper. Experts suggest that body language is more honest than verbal communication and gives a much stronger source of information than the spoken word. To illustrate this it might be useful to consider the reaction of an audience listening to a speaker talking about communication skills and yet failing to look at the audience while speaking. As one of the key aspects in good communication is maintaining eye contact, the non-verbal cues received by the audience in this situation may not match the content of the lecture. This is a key factor that must be considered.

    The speaker should of course face the audience and should aim, as far as possible, to maintain eye contact with that group. This may not be easy for the newcomer to lecturing but it does become easier with practice.

Other traits should be considered. For example, do not point at people, do not stand with arms folded, do not turn your back on the audience. All of these are distancing gestures. In addition any mannerisms that may be seen as irritating by your audience should be avoided. Twiddling with a curl of hair, for example, may be a mild mannerism but can be very irritating to members of an audience if it distracts them from the content of the presentation.

5. Ways of encouraging audience participation can be considered. Anecdotes can increase audience participation and change their role from a passive to an active one. They should, however, be used with caution for they can be distracting when factual material is being presented.

    If the speaker has the confidence, and opportunity allows, questioning the audience can increase participation and serve to sustain interest. This approach is perhaps only of use with smaller audiences.

There are many tricks of the trade adopted by teachers to maintain the interest of their audience. Such skills are seen as essential in teaching for there is evidence to suggest that when listening to lectures concentration cannot be sustained for a long period. Consequently it is useful to consider ways in which the key points of any lecture can be made clear to the audience. Although, with practice, public speakers can do much to enhance the liveliness of their verbal presentation and so retain interest, audio-visual aids also offer an excellent medium by which points can be clarified and audience concentration focused.

Audio-visual aids

In this modern world the scope and variety of audio-visual aids available is tremendous, ranging from the chalkboard through to computer technology. When presenting a lecture, however, speakers need to feel confident with any equipment used and this does, to some extent, limit the range of audio-visual aids that can be utilised by the newcomer to public speaking. Consequently the following discussion will only focus on a few of the more popular visual aids used. It should be stressed at the outset that audio-visual aids are of benefit only if they are used well. If speakers have any doubt about their ability to use them, they may be better advised to limit their use until more practised. However relevant or interesting a talk is, inappropriate use of visual aids can distract an audience in such a way as to spoil the reception of the information by the audience.

Chalkboard

The chalkboard has been a common sight in classrooms for many years and still remains a popular tool in teaching. Traditionally the term 'blackboard' is used, but as modern technology takes over and we have available white boards, on which coloured ink pens are used, different names will be used to describe a similar visual aid.

The advantages of using boards of any sort are that it allows the lecturer to note key points as they arise in the presentation, to indicate how issues are linked by illustration and to demonstrate factual material more clearly. Information noted on the board should be minimal with only key points noted. For example a researcher may use this medium to highlight a few key results following a research study. It is not correct use to attempt to write out a mini version of lecture notes.

The first disadvantage of using a board is that it requires a moderate amount of confidence on the part of the lecturer. Thinking about what to write at the same time as concentrating on what is being said can be quite a complex process.

If used inappropriately this tool can serve to alienate the speaker from the audience. First, it is difficult to write without the speaker turning their back on the audience. Secondly if the speaker is not able to write clearly and concisely the effort made to use the board may be wasted as the audience may cease to concentrate on what is being said, trying instead to translate the symbols on the board.

In relation to this last point chalkboards are generally only of use if speaking to fairly small groups for all members of the audience should be able to read what has been written without any difficulty. If speakers find themselves with a large group and with only this medium for illustration then they should make minimal use of the board and adjust the size of their writing to ensure that all of the audience can see what has been written. If in doubt, it is better to avoid using it.

Flipcharts

Flipcharts are a similar medium to chalkboards in that they can be used to place emphasis on specific points when presenting information. The charts can be prepared in advance if there are key areas that will be usefully highlighted on one large page. This medium is particularly useful for the speaker leading a session in which audience participation was required and they wished to note down ideas generated for future discussion. This approach may be quite well suited to a small discussion group.

Overhead projector

The overhead projector (OHP) is a very popular visual aid in classroom settings and lecture theatres. Consequently this is a useful tool for larger audiences as the size of the projection on a screen (or plain wall) can be adjusted to meet the size of the room in which the machine is located. In addition, as the speaker does not need to turn away from the audience to use the OHP they can concentrate on audience response more than is possible with a chalkboard.

The OHP has other advantages. Although it can be used in the same way as the chalkboard for noting key points, acetates for use can be prepared well in advance of the lecture. Prepared acetates can serve to give an instant *aide-mémoire* if the headings are related closely to the content of the lecture.

Also, it has been noted that a picture is worth a thousand words. A clear concise diagram can have a much stronger impact on the audience than a long, detailed explanation. Consequently this is particularly useful to researchers looking for ways to summarise findings.

A major disadvantage of using the OHP is that, as with all mechanical objects, it may break down at a crucial moment. If the speaker is not skilled in maintaining this equipment, and carrying out procedures such as changing light bulbs, it is useful to check if there will be technicians available to help and advise. However, to be prepared, if you are planning to use this tool, it is always as well to think in advance how you would present the lecture in case the equipment fails.

The second potential disadvantage of using an OHP relates to the preparation of the acetates. There are many complex techniques that can be used to enhance the quality of acetates, particularly with computer programs available specifically for that purpose. It will be useful to consider a few simple points:

1. Do not attempt to put too much information on the acetate. The impact of a few key words is stronger than a sheet filled with a lot of detailed information.
2. The size of the letters/figures used is important. If very small writing is used it may not be seen at the back of the room. There are no rigid rules to follow but letters should be at least 5 mm in size and it is better to print than to link letters. It is advisable to test your acetates for clarity on an OHP well before the lecture to allow time for improvement if necessary.
3. There·are a variety of pens available for preparing acetates by hand. Spirit-based pens tend to give a sharper finish to writing on acetates but are not as easy to clean off if a mistake is made. Water-based pens are easy to use but can be very easily smudged if the acetate gets damp. The choice of pens may be affected by what is available at the time of preparation.
4. Pens (and computer programs) offer a variety of colours and it is very tempting to use all colours when preparing acetates. For impact, however, it is better to use a limited range of only two or three colours as this is less distracting for the audience. Also there is a need to take care in the choice of colours used. Some, such as yellow, may seem appealing when preparing acetates but do not show up very well on the screen. Light colours may be better used for shading words or pictures to create visual impact.
5. Diagrams and pictures can be demonstrated well with acetates as long as they too are kept simple. If demonstrating research results, graphs or histograms can be transferred onto an acetate to provide a clear source of reference for the audience. More than one acetate can be used to 'build up' a picture by placing a second one on top of the first. Although a useful technique, it is important not to overdo this. Too many acetates may serve to confuse if the detail becomes too complex. Also the finished product may not be very clear as the light source will become diluted by the thickness of the acetates.
6. Cartoons are a useful way of giving impact to a message, or simply to introduce some variety into a presentation. These are easily traced from original pictures if using acetates. However, cartoons should be used sparingly. The occasional

picture can have a big impact, too many can be tedious for the audience and distract from the main theme of the presentation.

7.   Finally there are some general points in relation to using an OHP that should be briefly outlined. First, do practise using the OHP before an important lecture. It can be very irritating to an audience if the speaker is fumbling around trying to get the machine to work. In addition a speaker should be prepared to raise his or her voice if the OHP has a noisy fan system as some of the older models do.

It is important that the lecturer does not stand in front of the OHP when giving a presentation. If he or she does, all the hard work of preparation will be in vain for the audience will only see the outline of the speaker's body. Equally it is important not to cover the acetate with a hand when displaying information on the OHP, firstly because it is very distracting and, secondly, because if the speaker is very nervous when talking, the shaking hand will be well magnified for all to see. It is far better to use a small object such as a pencil to emphasise a word on your acetate. If this is done, the lecturer can rest his or her hand on the side of the machine – an approach that can help reduce tremor.

Gradual exposure of information on an OHP is a useful way of focusing audience attention. This is easily done by covering the key point with paper and uncovering the words one at a time.

Finally, avoid looking into the light of the OHP as this can be blinding to the speaker and take concentration away from the audience.

Practising beforehand allows the speaker to check these points and also gives an opportunity to see if acetates are clear and easy to read when positioned on the OHP. Familiarity with working with prepared acetates will help increase confidence when giving a lecture.

Slides

In a large audience the use of slides offers a very effective means of ensuring that everybody can see information. If slides are to be used it is important that this is considered well in advance because they do take some time to prepare.

As with acetates the amount of information on a slide should be kept to a minimum although it is possible to put some quite complex tables on for reference purposes. When presenting research findings issues related to presentation of tables and graphs in Chapter 10 should be considered, for the same principles apply when using slides.

Slides can be used for written statements and for pictorial demonstration. If, for any reason pictures of individuals are to be included in a presentation, speakers should ensure that specific permission to use that material has been given and that, where necessary, confidentiality is maintained. For example if a nurse had undertaken a study into a new treatment for pressure sores she may want to show a picture of a patient before and after that treatment. She would need to get that patient's permission to exhibit the picture and may need to deface it to protect the patient's identity.

There is of course only value in showing pictures if they demonstrate what it is you want them to show. Poor quality slides are better not used.

The disadvantage in using slides is coping with the technology. It may give the speaker more confidence if he or she has placed the slides in the projector for at least he or she will then know that they are in the right order and position in the projector. This will also give an opportunity to practise changing slides and adjusting lighting. It is advisable to do this before the presentation.

Using computers to enhance presentations

The development of multimedia technology is such that complex presentations allowing the integration of OHP information, picture slides and even video can now be incorporated into programmes for presentation at conferences. If you have such facilities available to you and wish to use them the important point is, as above, to practise with the technology before your presentation. A good presentation using such technology is most impressive; if it goes wrong it tends to do so in a big way – or at least it seems like a big way when you are trying to adjust your programme in front of an audience!

Hand-outs

Hand-outs which give additional information can be very useful to the audience but as they can be quite costly it is important to consider carefully whether the use is appropriate. If hand-outs are used the lecturer should consider carefully when they will be circulated. If they have been designed to save the audience taking any notes it is no good circulating them at the end of the lecture after the audience has been busily writing down everything that has been said. Alternatively, if the information on the hand-out is supplementary to the talk then it would be appropriate to circulate it when the lecture is finished. The audience should be told if there is a hand-out available and where and when it will be circulated. Again quality of presentation is an important point in preparing hand-outs.

Poster displays

It is quite a common practice in conferences for a room to be set aside for poster displays. A poster display is not an aid to help in a presentation of a lecture, rather it is an alternative medium by which research findings can be shared with colleagues. The skill required for presentation in this way incorporates both written and presentation skills. The emphasis is on the posters which should convey the information in a clear and unambiguous way. If summarising a research project for a poster display then the same guidelines as those given for writing a research report apply. Key points should be specifically highlighted to give instant visual impact to the reader and, in relation to this, other information should be kept to a minimum. The idea is to give a concise overview of the subject in such a way that it is appealing to the eye. Supplementary material can be made available in the form of hand-outs if necessary. As with verbal presentations noted above, the development of computing technology is such that people who present posters in conference can give a very professional finish with appropriate help and guidance. If a researcher was asked to do a poster display of his or her work then the organiser would assume that he or she would be available to talk to people interested in the study and results. So, although this method of presentation may not be as threatening as giving a lecture, it still requires an ability to communicate well.

The audio-visual aids discussed above are those most commonly used in seminars of conferences where research findings are presented. The use and abuse of audio-visual aids is a subject worthy of much more detailed exploration but space has allowed only an overview in this text. Confidence with this equipment only comes with practice and the skills can be developed with experience of presenting information. There are people who will be able to help and advise about preparing material for presentation in lectures, for example an audio-visual technician in a medical illustration department in a hospital or in a university, a teacher, or simply a colleague who has had some experience of lecturing. A practitioner who has developed a research study and is in a position to share knowledge with colleagues will find that by making use of these resources they help facilitate a good quality presentation.

ACTIVITY _____

- Identify an area of research you would like to develop (use your examples from earlier chapters if you wish).
- Refer to Figure 11.1 and jot down a few notes under each heading to indicate the process you would go through if you were to develop this into a full research proposal.

Summary

This chapter has explored the writing and presentation skills required for the final stages of the research process. Such skills are necessary to complete the research process. Moreover they represent the first stage of research dissemination which will be considered further in the next chapter.

Further reading

Burnard, P. (1995) *Writing for Health*, Chapman & Hall, London.
Clancy, J. and Ballard, B. (1983) *How to Write Essays. A Practical Guide for Students*, Longman, Cheshire, Melbourne.

Gowers, E. (1987) *The Complete Plain Words*, revised by S. Greenbaum and J. Whitcut, Penguin, Harmondsworth.
Jay, A. (1985) *Effective Presentation: The Communication of Ideas by Words and Visual Aids*, BIM (British Institute of Management), London.
Philips, L.R.F. (1986) *A Clinician's Guide to the Critique and Utilisation of Nursing Research*, Appleton Century Crofts, Connecticut.

See also: 'Writing and Research', *Nurse Researcher*, vol. 2, no. 1, September (1993).

12   Using research in clinical practice

In this text the research process has been traced from the point of developing an idea through to the processes of writing and presenting research findings. This last step is the beginning of the stage of 'dissemination' in research. This is important for research must be available if we are to consider the principles of implementing research into practice, a step that may be considered the final stage of the research process (see Figure 12.1). In this chapter we will consider in the last two phases of the research process:

1. Disseminating research findings.
2. Implementing research in practice.

Disseminating research findings

Unless the results of research are shared it is unlikely that research-based practice will advance much further. From this perspective there is a need to consider who is responsible for disseminating research findings and ways in which this may be facilitated.

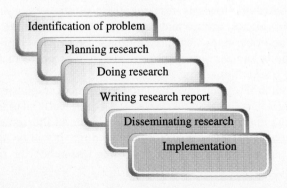

Figure 12.1 The stages of the research process.

Who is responsible for disseminating research?

Dissemination of research activity is a major concern of a number of organisations as illustrated in Figure 12.2. Broadly this can be traced through management, education and professional routes, all of which have a two-way relationship with those responsible for the direct management of clinical practice.

In recent years in the United Kingdom the Department of Health has identified R&D as a major priority in health care management. This in turn has resulted in a cascade of R&D management through regional centres to local clinical units. The impact of the NHS R&D strategy is increasingly evident in health care as it has contributed towards identifying a range of discrepancies in the utilisation of research in health care and illustrated the tendency for practice in a ritualistic rather than a research-based way in many areas of health care. In addition it has identified a number of areas where there is insufficient research available to inform practice. Consequently two major strands of activity have emerged with emphasis on both research and development of practice based on research. First an active research programme of health care research into areas of practice has been established. Linked with this, systems for disseminating research findings have been implemented, and the Cochrane Centre and York Centre for Reviews and Dissemination play a major role in undertaking critical reviews of the range of research literature of research completed in health care to help speed up the process of dissemination to practitioners.

Other organisations interested in developing and disseminating research-based activity include the education sector, primarily universities. A key feature of the NHS R&D strategy is that it has encouraged collaborative working between the NHS and the education sector in the development of research for clinical practice. Universities contribute to research dissemination at different levels, first in developing research activity, and secondly in disseminating research findings through teaching, publishing research findings in academic journals and through conferences. Finally, in recent years, universities have taken a more active interest in the implementation of research into practice and there has been an increase in the range of posts which involve practitioners in joint working between clinical posts and the university.

The last route identified in Figure 12.2 is the professional route. Professional organisations contribute towards research dissemination in a number of ways including specialist interest groups and networks for supporting the dissemination of information. In addition many academic journals are actively supported by professional organisations and the publication of research, as noted in Chapter 11, is a major forum for research dissemination.

At an individual professional level all practitioners hold responsibility for ensuring that their practice is based on sound knowledge. Consequently all practitioners should be involved in the dissemination of research findings. As illustrated in Figure 12.2 there are a number of ways in which this can be done. It will be useful to consider this further in relation to the specific roles of the researcher, the manager and the teacher in nursing.

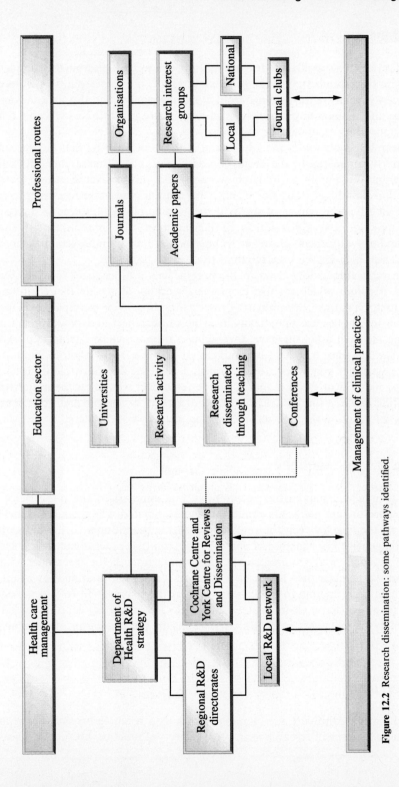

Figure 12.2 Research dissemination: some pathways identified.

The researcher

Planning for research should include consideration of how findings from the completed study should be disseminated to the profession. This is important not only from the point of view of sharing the findings from a specific project but also as a means of stimulating and maintaining the interest of health care practitioners who have not had the opportunity to undertake research.

The researcher is obviously the key person in terms of ensuring that any research findings are disseminated to the profession. However, not all researchers in health care are employed purely as research workers and this has implications for the dissemination of findings. Practitioners may, for example, undertake research projects as part of an advanced course of study. If they are employed full time in a clinical post they may not be in a position to go out and meet other practitioners to share research findings with them. However willing they are, their employers may not be able to release them for the time required to do this effectively.

The research method adopted may play a part in facilitating feedback to professional colleagues. Methods which involve researchers working alongside their colleagues can be a useful means of disseminating research findings. For example participant observation techniques are one means by which researchers and practitioners can work alongside each other, perhaps developing a rapport which facilitates dissemination of findings once the study is complete. Action research is another method in which the researcher may work closely with staff involved the study (see Chapter 6).

Although in an ideal world it should be the researcher who takes the initiative in disseminating research knowledge, this may not always be feasible and other means of filtering information through to practitioners need to be considered.

The health care manager

In a world in which managerial accountability is emphasised the importance of research to health care managers cannot be underestimated. The manager is ideally placed to be the link between the researcher and the practitioner. If the researcher shares findings with one member of clinical staff then that practitioner may effect a change in practice as appropriate within his or her unit. If the researcher shares findings with a manager then the cascade effect of sharing information may result in the dissemination of findings to several units that are the responsibility of the manager. It should be noted that a clear impact of the NHS R&D strategy is to increase the accountability of managers in health care to ensure the utilisation of research in practice.

Education staff

The educators in health care are commonly seen as a resource for knowledge and this as true in the area of research as in other aspects of practice. Lecturers in health care have responsibility for sharing research knowledge with two groups, students and practitioners working in clinical areas. It is therefore critical that lecturers are themselves well prepared to present research knowledge to their students. This role is crucial when considering the dissemination of research findings. The impact of a lively, well-prepared lecture or discussion on the subject of research has the potential to affect a critical review of practice in many areas.

Quite commonly the lecturer carries a lot of responsibility for sustaining an interest in research once it has been generated. If the style of professional education encourages questioning and demands that the knowledge base of practice is research based then it is highly likely that this approach will stay with the student throughout his or her career in health care. Once a research-based approach to education has been adopted it is important to maintain the initiative and not to revert to traditional patterns of education. One of the benefits of moving education for health care practitioners into the universities is that for many, it means they will be exposed to a research-orientated culture – a culture that was not the case in many NHS-based schools where the emphasis was on training to care (see Chapter 2).

How can research findings be disseminated?

There are several ways in which research findings can be disseminated to practitioners and for the purpose of clarity they will be discussed under separate headings.

Returning information to the research site

When researchers seek permission to undertake research they commonly make a promise to let those people who have participated in the study know of the results as soon as they are made available. This can be a very useful way of sharing research findings; the interest of participants is likely to be high because of personal involvement in the research. An additional benefit is that insight gained from participants after the event may be useful to the researcher in planning future studies. For example the sample group may wish to make observations about their perception of research methods used in the study. It is important that researchers recognise these factors and ensure that they share their findings through these channels.

Another reason why this is important is in considering the interests of future studies being undertaken within that environment. If staff receive promises of feedback from researchers, and then these promises are not met, staff will be less likely to co-operate with future researchers looking for permission to undertake studies in that area.

Publishing research findings

As noted in Chapter 11 one of the most obvious ways to share research findings is to ensure that the results are published and shared with as many people as possible.

This may seem very obvious but it can cause difficulty in practice for several reasons. Firstly, writing does take quite a long time and newcomers to research often underestimate the time it will take them to prepare their work for publication. A useful guide for researchers to work to is that the time allowed for writing a report should represent about a third of the total time allowed for the whole research project. If the time taken for material to be published is added to this it can be seen that there is a long time span between beginning a research project and publication.

This leads to the second problem which is that there are only a limited number of national and international journals that publish research. As a result of this the time taken for publication can be variable, extending in some instances to a couple of years. The immediate relevance of a research project may be lost in a long time lapse such as this, so researchers need to consider other ways of disseminating their findings.

In considering quicker ways in which to communicate their findings than the national publication process researchers might be able to identify whether there are any local journals that could be used to disseminate information to staff who might have particular interest in the research. For example, a lot of NHS trusts have small journals for local news and comments and the editors of these are commonly looking for material.

Study days and conferences

Study days and conferences provide a very useful medium for sharing experiences and consequently offer one of the commonest routes for disseminating research findings. These forums are not confined to a select group of nurse researchers. One of the positive developments of post basic courses in professional education today is that students who have undertaken research studies will frequently report their findings in a locally arranged study day. Such an approach has the benefit of identifying issues specifically related to the locality and can therefore be a useful means of increasing research awareness.

Research interest groups

Research interest groups provide a means by which those people interested in research can share experiences. Whilst providing a forum for the dissemination of findings from research studies these groups also offer a resource for those people undertaking research. Local research interest groups may be identified within a health care unit. In addition there are national research interest groups commonly associated with the professional organisations for health care.

Research appreciation courses

Research courses are another common way in which information can be disseminated. Health care practitioners undertaking the course will become increasingly aware of research as the programme develops. In addition to this colleagues may express an interest and make enquiries about the content of the course. This may ultimately motivate others to undertake research studies themselves.

Linked with this is the increasing flexibility of educational approaches. For example, distance learning is a useful means of facilitating an educational opportunity for nurses and health care practitioners. This approach can be utilised regardless of irregular working hours and other difficulties that sometimes hinder practitioners wishing to undertake advanced study. Such approaches have been adopted by some educational centres as a means of developing research knowledge. Further details relating to distance learning packages can be obtained from the organisations in the further reading section at the end of this chapter.

Using research in practice

Research, quite commonly, generates more questions than answers. Thus health care practitioners seeking information to help them in their work may still find themselves faced with a number of questions rather than a clearly defined action plan for using research in practice.

A criticism that could be directed at experimental research, for example, may be that the studies themselves are carried out in such a manner that they do not reflect the day-to-day practices of health care. Researchers are able to manipulate the variables in a way that may be beyond the control of practitioners. For example, there is a lot of research work undertaken into communication in patient care in hospital. Depending upon the research design the researcher may have been able to control the time spent in communicating with the patients. Consequently, although the result of such a study may demonstrate the importance of spending time communicating with patients, the nurse or other health care worker working in busy health care units may not be able to utilise the research for the simple reason that the unit has staff shortages. The staff in the ward or unit may have less time available to them than that allocated to patient/client communication by the researcher.

However, the practitioner can still use the research in a constructive way, for example by using the research findings to make a case for more staff in the unit and therefore work towards creating the right environment in which these research findings can be utilised. Consequently, although at the outset some research may be seen to reflect an ideal environment, it can still have utility value in practice.

Implementing research findings

Given the potential difficulties linked with using research in practice there is a need to consider how health care practitioners can go about implementing research in practice. If this is to be achieved it would appear that there are several areas that need to be addressed. The first is that, as indicated above, if research is to be implemented it needs to be *available* to practitioners. In the local setting therefore it

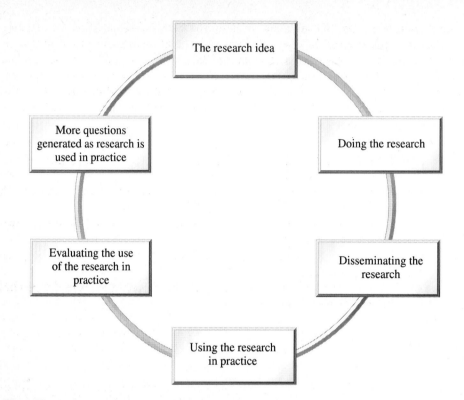

Figure 12.3 From research idea to practice: a cyclical process.

is important that practitioners review ways in which they can receive such information, perhaps referring to the ways indicated in Figure 12.2.

The next critical point is that practitioners need the *knowledge* to be able to understand the research process. As indicated in Chapter 2 one of the key factors influencing research awareness is knowledge about research – if practitioners have little insight into research processes they are not in a position to utilise this. This is a critical point for unless there is sufficient knowledge about the research processes, research may be inappropriately utilised. A key factor practitioners learn on programmes educating them about research is that not all published research is good research; it is essential that they have the knowledge to make the distinction between poor and good research before proceeding.

Assuming practitioners have the necessary knowledge base the next issue is the need to ensure there is a *receptive environment* in which practitioners are prepared to challenge practices that have become 'rituals' or traditions in the workplace (see Chapters 2 and 5). This brings the debate around to *supportive managerial structures* that will facilitate processes of change and a knowledge of how change processes work in complex health care organisations.

Linked with the process of implementing change is the need to consider whether any changes in practice developed out of research are having an impact. It is interesting to note that whilst many health care professionals are still struggling with the ideas inherent in getting research used in practice, at a national level a question that is now being asked is 'how effective is the care that is being offered?'. This means that introducing research into practice remains only one step in a far more complex process of evaluating the outcomes of health care provision as illustrated in Figure 12.3. The skills required to evaluate the impact of care based on research include those research skills outlined in this book.

ACTIVITY _____

- Review your own work environment and consider ways in which research is disseminated.
- List the factors that may enhance the utilisation of research in your own area of practice.
- List the factors that may impede the utilisation of research in your own area of practice.
- Consider what action you could take to help increase the research profiles of your own area of work.

Summary

This chapter has briefly addressed disseminating and implementing research findings in practice. This brings the research process full circle from original idea to the impact on practice. If you refer back to the beginning of this text you will note a key word in research is 'why'. Perhaps you will have realised by now that this is a question to which the range of answers may be inconclusive and that an end point of research is an elusive concept. Whilst change based on research findings may help improve aspects of care it is also likely that it will generate more 'why' questions. As the knowledge base increases then so too does the search for more knowledge. The resolution of one set of problems by the utilisation of research findings serves to generate the next set of questions that require an answer! To be able to respond to the questions that arise you need a clear understanding of the research process and a good insight into the managerial strategies necessary to facilitate the process of change required to implement those findings in practice. In so doing remember you are not alone – there are many people seeking to learn these skills and many others willing to help them do so, so please ask for help if you need it.

Further reading

Baker, M. and Kirk, S. (Eds) (1995) *Research and Development for the NHS: Evidence, Evaluation and Effectiveness*, NAHAT, Radcliffe Medical Press, Oxford.

Carnwell, R. (1997) *Evaluative Research Methodology in Nursing and Health Care*, Open Learning Foundation/Churchill Livingstone, Edinburgh.

Clark, J. and Copcutt, L. (1996) *Management for Nurses and Health Care Professionals*, Churchill Livingstone, Edinburgh.

Crabtree, B. F., Miller, W. L., Addison, R. B., Gilchrist, V. J. and Kuzel, A. (1994) *Exploring Collaborative Research in Primary Care*, Sage, London.

Department of Health (1991) *Research for Health A Research & Development Strategy for the NHS*, Department of Health, London Peckham M.

Department of Health (1993) *Report of the Taskforce on the Strategy for Research in Nursing, Midwifery and Health Visiting*, Department of Health, London Webb A.

Department of Health (1995) *Methods to Promote the Implementation of Research Findings in the NHS – Priorities for Evaluation*, Department of Health, London.

Dunn, E., Norton, P. G., Stewart, M., Tudiver, F. and Bass, M. J. (1994) *Conducting Research in the Practice Setting*, Sage, London.

Hunt, J. (1981) 'Indicators for nursing practice: The use of research findings', *Journal of Advanced Nursing*, vol. 6, no. 3, pp. 189–194.

Hunt, J. (1996) 'Barriers to research utilisation', *Journal of Advanced Nursing*, vol. 23, pp. 423–425.

McIntosh, J. (1995) 'Barriers to research implementation', *Nurse Researcher*, vol. 2, no. 4, pp. 83–91.

Reed, J. and Proctor, S. (Eds) (1995) *Practitioner Research in Health Care: The Inside Story*, Chapman & Hall, London.

Therapy Profession Research Group (1994) *Research and Development in Occupational Therapy, Physiotherapy and Speech and Language Therapy. A Position Statement*, Department of Health, London.

Refer also to Open/Distant Learning programmes available from: the Open University, School of Health and Social Welfare, Walton Hall, Milton Keynes MK7 6AA; Royal College of Nursing, Institute of Advanced Education, 20 Cavendish Square, London W1M 0AB; the University of the South Bank, Distance Learning Centre, 103 Borough Road, London SE1 0AA; Macmillan Open Learning, Porters South, 4 Crinan Street, London N1 9XW; the Open Learning Foundation/Churchill Livingstone, Healthcare Active Learning Series, 3 Devonshire Street, London W1N 2BA.

Glossary

Action research An approach to research that adopts the principles of the problem-solving cycle of assessment, planning implementation and evaluation.

Analysis The process of interpreting **data** or information gathered in the research study.

Anthropological research The study of culture, people in social, institutional and social settings (see **ethnography**).

Bias Any influence that may distort the findings of a research study.

Blind trial A design used in experimental research in which the participants do not know what treatment they are receiving (see also **double blind trial**).

Bracketing A process used in qualitative research by which a researcher endeavours to distance his or her personal experiences to avoid bias when collecting data from an individual.

Case study An approach to research in which the researcher focuses on a single 'case' to study a particular phenomenon. The 'case' may be an individual, a group or an institution.

Cause and effect A term commonly used in the context of developing a hypothesis which tests cause and effect.

CD-ROM Refers to 'compact disc, read only memory' to describe computerised library indexes of published articles and books.

Central tendency A statistical term used to describe the 'central' scores in the distribution of a set of figures. Measures of central tendency include the **mean**, **median** and **mode**.

Clinical trial A term used to refer to research studies that employ experimental methods to study the impact of new clinical treatment such as drugs or techniques of care.

Closed question A question with a fixed range of mutually exclusive responses (e.g. 'yes' or 'no' or 'don't know'). Contrasts with **open question**.

Coding A process used in qualitative data analysis to identify common words or themes that recur in the data.

Compliance Used in research to indicate the extent to which respondents participate in a research study. Researchers seek to design studies in such a way that will reduce non-compliance (non-participation) in the research.

Concept An idea or notion to explain some commonly recognised phenomenon.

Conceptual framework A group of concepts linked together by propositions – may be referred to as a theoretical model.

Condition The situation under which participants are being studied.

Confounding variable A variable that varies systematically with the independent variable and so provides an alternative explanation for any effects on the dependent variable that are observed.

Constant error Any source of error which distorts or biases the results of research study in a constant reliable way.

Construct validity The level to which a research instrument measures the underlying construct or theory.

Content analysis The process of analysing **data** presented in words rather than figures (words generated through interviews, open-ended questions or field notes in qualitative research design).

Content validity An indicator of how well the content of a research instrument measures the phenomena or attributes on which the conclusions are to be based.

Control A concept used in **experimental research design** which indicates some control over the study by eliminating influences on the **dependent variable** other than those being manipulated by the researcher in the **independent variable**.

Control group A group of subjects in an experimental study who are not exposed to the **independent variable (IV)** but contribute to the study by participating in measures of the dependent variable enables the impact of the IV on the **experimental group** to be compared.

Convenience sample A sample selected on the basis of accessibility to the researcher rather than using **random sample** procedures.

Correlation A situation in which a variation in one variable is associated with a variation in another (see **Positive correlation, Negative correlation, Correlation coefficient**).

Correlation coefficient A measure used to describe the extent of the relationship between two variables in a correlational statistical test.

Correlational design A research method which aims to describe the relationship between naturally occurring variables.

Criterion-related validity Examines how well a research instrument correlates with other external measures of the same concept.

Crossover design An experimental research design in which two treatment conditions (e.g. placebo and independent variable) are sequenced in differing order to avoid risk of **Hawthorne effect** and **order effect**. Repeated measures are used throughout the study.

Data A term used to refer to information collected in a research study. This may be in words (**qualitative research methods**) or in numerical form (in **quantitative research methods**).

Data collection techniques Refers to the approaches used to collect data and may include **questionnaires, interviews, observation**, diaries, etc.

Deductive reasoning This involves using a known idea or theory and applying it to a different situation (see also **inductive reasoning**).

Dependent variable (DV) The variable within an hypothesis which is affected by the **independent variable** when stating an hypothesis.

Descriptive design An approach to research in which there is no attempt to control or manipulate **variables** and the researcher describes what is observed (see **non-experimental research**).

Descriptive statistics A type of statistics used to summarise data in descriptive research design (see also **inferential statistics**).

Different subject design An experimental research design in which each group takes part in the study by participating in one **condition** or treatment only.

Double blind trial A procedure used in experimental design to ensure that neither the participants nor the researcher know to which treatment condition a particular individual has been assigned.

Emic Refers to the perspective of the person being studied which is paramount in the analysis of data.

Empirical research Refers to research that uses forms of observation using the senses. Generally used in the context of scientific approach to research.

Epistemology The study of knowledge.

Ethnography A research approach in which the researcher seeks to understand human behaviour from the perspective of the individual in a given culture. Influenced by **anthropological research**.

Etic The perspective and insights of the observer influences the interpretation of data.

Evaluation research A research method which attempts to establish the value of a programme (for example, a programme of health care). The value is determined by whether or not the programme achieves its goals or meets the needs of users of the programme.

Event sampling A sampling technique used in observation techniques of data collection to focus the observation on the event as it occurs. Contrasts with **time sampling**.

Experimental design An approach to research in an attempt to look for **cause and effect**. The researcher **controls** the **independent variable** (experimental variable) and measures the effect on the **dependent variable**.

Experimental group A set of participants or subjects in a research study who are exposed to the independent variable (treatment or **condition**) being examined.

Experimental hypothesis The **hypothesis** stated in **experimental design**.

Experimental variable A term used to describe the independent variable manipulated by the researcher.

Experimenter bias effects Refers to any bias introduced by the researcher (experimenter) that may influence the results of a study.

Exploratory research Describes a research approach in which researchers are beginning to explore a specific phenomenon. Commonly used with **descriptive design**.

Extraneous variable Refers to any variable other than the independent variable which may influence the effect on the dependent variable to be measured.

Face validity This is a judgement of whether, on the 'face of it' the research instrument appears to measure what it is supposed to measure.

Feminist research An approach to research which considers the gender perspective.

Field notes The notes kept by a researcher undertaking an observation study 'in the field', i.e. the natural setting.

Focus group interview An interview technique in which a group of individuals may be interviewed simultaneously.

Forced choice questions An approach used in structured questionnaires in which the respondent is limited to a range of responses, thus the choice is forced.

Generalisability Refers to the extent to which the findings from a sample can be applied (generalised) to the **population** from which the sample was taken.

Grounded theory An approach to research in which the aim is to collect and analyse qualitative data with the intention of developing a theory which is 'grounded' in the data.

Hard data A term sometimes used for data that can be measured and quantified.

Hawthorne effect A phenomenon observed in research studies in which participant behaviour changes as a result of being observed (also referred to as the **placebo effect**).

Historical research The study of past events. Uses memories, record reviews and the principles of qualitative research design to analyse data.

Hypothesis (H_1) A statement of a relationship between two or more **variables**, the **independent variable (IV)** and the **dependent variable (DV)** (see also **null hypothesis**).

Independent variable (IV) The **variable** within a hypothesis which can be manipulated by the researcher to determine the effect on the **dependent variable**.

Inductive reasoning The use of observations to formulate an idea or theory rather than taking known ideas or theories.

Inferential statistics The type of statistical tests that are used to infer whether the observations in the sample studied are likely to occur in a larger population.

Instruments Refers to the 'tools' of data collection in research, e.g. questionnaires, interview, observation schedule or checklists.

Internal consistency Relates to the reliability of a research instrument in terms of the extent to which all components of the instrument are measuring the same attributes.

Interpretative research A term used to describe some approaches to qualitative research.

Interval data Data which can be measured on a scale where the distance or interval between each point is identical.

Interview An approach used in research in which the researcher collects data by face-to-face contact with the subject being studied. May be used with individuals or groups.

Interview schedule The research instrument (questionnaire or prompts) used to structure the interview.

Likert scale A five-point scale commonly used in questionnaires to measure attitudes to a given phenomena.

Literature critique A critical review of research material that uses knowledge of research methodology to judge the merits or otherwise of a piece of reported research.

Literature review A critical review of a range of literature relating to an area of interest.

Literature search The process of finding published literature relating to an area of research.

Manipulation A process used in experimental studies to research will manipulate the **independent variable** to see the effect on the **dependent variable**.

Mann–Whitney *U* test A non-parametric statistical test used to see whether there are significant differences between two sets of data which have come from two different sets of subjects.

Matched subject design A research design used in experimental research in which two or more groups of subjects are matched on factors that could bias the results.

Mean A measure of **central tendency** used to identify the average score in a set of figures. Classed as a **descriptive statistic**.

Median A measure of **central tendency** in a set of figures by identifying the score which falls exactly in the middle of a set of figures. Classed as a **descriptive statistic**.

Meta-analysis Combining a critique of methodology and the results from several studies to determine the collective view.

Mode A measure of **central tendency** used to describe the most frequently occurring number in a set of figures. Classed as a **descriptive statistic**.

Negative correlation Used to describe the result of **correlation** research in which an increase in the score of one **variable** is associated with a decrease in the other.

NHS UK National Health Service.

Nominal data Data that can be placed in named categories.

Non-experimental research A term sometimes used to describe a research approach that does not involve manipulation, control or randomisation. May be used interchangeably with **descriptive** research.

Non-parametric tests A type of statistical test which does not rely on a set of parameters. These type of tests are not as sensitive as **parametric tests**.

Non-participant observation See **observation**.

Non-probability sampling An approach to sampling which does not involve the principles of random sampling.

Normal distribution Refers to a distribution of data that is symmetrical and thus when presented in graph form shows a bell shape.

Null hypothesis A hypothesis written in such a way as to indicate that there is no relationship between the **independent variable** and the **dependent variable**. Required for statistical testing procedures (see also **hypothesis**).

Observation A research technique in which a researcher observes subjects in order to gather data. May range from 'participation' to 'non-participation' techniques. Also used in reference to general observations made in **empirical research** studies.

One-tailed hypothesis test A hypothesis in which only one outcome is predicted (see also **two-tailed hypothesis test**).

Open question A question which gives the respondent the scope to develop an individual response in their own words. Is used in qualitative research designs and contrasts with **closed questions**.

Opportunistic sampling An approach to sampling used in qualitative research when the researcher selects a sample as the opportunity presents using the principles of **purposive/ theoretical sampling** to identify the sample.

Order effect A measurable change in participants in an experimental study that may result from their experiencing one treatment condition before another (see **crossover design** and **placebo effect**).

Ordinal data Data allocated to named categories that may be 'ordered', for example from least to strongest (e.g. strongly agree to disagree).

Parallel form Refers to a type of testing for reliability in which the findings for the research instrument undergoing development are compared with an established format.

Parametric test A type of statistical test that relies on the presence of certain conditions or parameters in order to carry out a test of this kind (see **non-parametric tests**).

Participant observation See **observation**.

Participants Describes the people involved in a research study (see **respondents** and **subjects**).

Phenomenology An approach to research which emphasises and seeks to explore the real life experience of the individual (influenced by philosophical reasoning).

Pilot study A small-scale test of a **research design** completed before the main study to enable a researcher to test whether the design will work.

Placebo An inactive substance or form of treatment used in experimental research design (e.g. drug trials) to compare with the effect of the independent variable (the active treatment) on the dependent variable.

Placebo effect A phenomenon observed in research studies in which participant behaviour changes as a result of being observed (also referred to as the **Hawthorne effect**).

Population The entire set of subjects in a given group that form the focus of a study. The **sample** is drawn from the population.

Positive correlation The result of **correlation** research in which an increase in the score of one variable is associated with an increased score in the other variable.

Positivist research Refers to research in the scientific tradition that involves quantification of data.

Post-test The stage of data collection completed after the administration of the independent variable in experimental research designs (see **pre-test**).

Pre-test This has two meanings. The first is as part of experimental design – the first stage of data collection to establish baseline data. The other is when it is used as a trial run to test instruments when developing a research study – the term is sometimes used when the study is too small to undertake a pilot study.

Probability (*p*) See **significance level**.

Probability sampling An approach to sampling which involves the principles of random sampling.

Prospective study An approach in which a relationship between variables is predicted and data collected as time progresses to determine if assumptions are correct (contrasts with **retrospective study**).

Purposive sample A sampling technique used in qualitative research in which the researcher chooses the sample on the basis of known characteristics or experiences.

Qualitative research methods Term used to describe research methods which collect and analyse non-numerical **data**. Contrasts with **quantitative research methods**.

Quantitative research methods Term used to describe research methods which collect data which can be analysed numerically. Contrasts with **qualitative research methods**.

Questionnaire A research instrument or 'tool' for data collection in research. May contain **closed** and/or **open questions**.

R&D Research and development.

Random error An error which obscures the results of the **independent variable** on the dependent variable in experimental research. Produced by variation of **extraneous variable** or inaccuracy of measurement.

Random sample A sampling procedure which ensures each member of the **population** being studied has an equal chance of being selected.

Range A measure used in **descriptive statistics** to indicate the difference between the highest and lowest scores in a set of figures.

Rank A numerical value given to an observation denoting its relative order in a set of data.

Ranking scales An approach to data collection used in quantitative research in which respondents are asked to rank options from 'least' to 'most' on the scale.

Related *t* test A parametric statistical test used for matched subject or same subject design.

Reliability The extent to which a research instrument/procedure produces the same results when tested under consistent conditions.

Replication study A study that replicates another. More commonly used in quantitative research approaches where the research design is sufficiently described to enable replication to occur.

Research design The overall plan for **data** collection and **analysis** in a research study.

Research instrument Refers to the 'tool' used for data collection, for example may be questionnaire, an interview schedule, an observation schedule or a checklist.

Research process The procedures involved when implementing the **research design**.

Research proposal The plan used to establish the framework for the research study.

Research question The question or problem that underpins a research study. May be developed into aims/objectives or a hypothesis.

Research supervisor A person who has greater experience of research and acts in the capacity as guide or mentor to someone undertaking a research study.

Research team Refers to a group of people working on a single research project.

Respondents People who participate in a research study by responding to questions asked. May be used interchangeably with '**subjects**' or **sample** in a research report.

Retrospective study Data collected after the event, therefore retrospective (contrasts with **prospective study**).

Same subject design An approach used in experimental research design in which each subject is tested on two or more occasions (for example, a pre- and post-test). Contrasts with **different subject design**.

Sample A small group drawn from a larger **population**. Different approaches to sampling include random, purposive, opportunistic convenience samples, etc.

Saturation A term used to describe the point at which the researcher gathering and analysing qualitative data feels no new categories are emerging in the analysis.

Scientific approach A term generally used to refer to research that reflect experimental approaches to data collection and analysis.

Semi-structured interview An approach to interview using a semi-structured interview schedule or questionnaire.

Significance level The **probability (*p*)** of an error occurring in the results of a study as a result of random error or chance.

Snowball sampling A sampling technique used in qualitative research in which researchers ask respondents to identify any other people who might fit the sampling requirement, thus the sample grows. (Arises from **opportunistic sampling**.)

Soft data A term sometimes used for data that are not quantified in numerical terms therefore refers to data generated by qualitative research design.

Spearman correlation test A non-parametric statistical test used to detect if there is any relationship between two variables.

Standard deviation (SD) A measure of the degree of variability of a set of scores. Indicates how much a set of figures is dispersed from the mean score.

Stratified sample A technique in which **random sampling** may be used to select people from two or more strata of the **population** independently.

Structured interview An approach to interviewing in research using a structured interview schedule or questionnaire.

Structured questionnaire A type of questionnaire design which consists of **closed questions** which give it a high level of structure (contrasts with semi-structured questionnaire which may contain more **open questions**).

Subjects The **sample** in a research study. See also **respondents**.

Survey A research method involved in the collection of **descriptive** data from a large number of respondents. Commonly uses **questionnaire** and/or **interview** technique of **data collection**.

Telephone interviews An approach used in interview techniques of data collection in which, rather than a face-to-face meeting, interviews are conducted over the telephone.

Test–retest reliability A form of reliability testing in which a research instrument that is being developed is administered on two separate occasions to the same subject with view to identifying whether responses are consistent.

Theoretical sampling An approach used in sampling in **grounded theory** in which the sampling technique is based on the concepts that have theoretical relevance to the evolving theory.

Theory An abstract generalisation indicating relationship between concepts and constructs.

Time sampling An approach to observation research in which the researcher undertakes observation in blocks of time (contrasts with **event sampling**).

Tools (of research) A word sometimes used to describe the instruments used for data collection (e.g. questionnaires, interview/observation schedules/checklists).

Transcribing data To transcribe means to write out fully the qualitative data collected.

Triangulation The use of more than one method of collecting or interpreting data.

Two-tailed hypothesis A hypothesis statement that has two possible outcomes (see also **One-tailed hypothesis**).

Unrelated *t* test A parametric statistical test used for different subject design.

Validity The extent to which a research tool measures what it is supposed to measure.

Variable The characteristics or features of the objects or people in a research study (see also **independent variable** and **dependent variable**).

Visual analogue scale A measure that can be used in questionnaires to enable respondents to indicate strength of feeling on a line drawing.

Wilcoxon signed ranks test A non-parametric statistical test used to see whether there are significant differences between two sets of data from a **same** or **matched subject design**.

Index

201